THE CHALLENGE TO CHANGE

A volume in the series
The Culture and Politics of Health Care Work
edited by Suzanne Gordon and Sioban Nelson

A list of titles in this series is available at www.cornellpress.cornell.edu

THE CHALLENGE
TO CHANGE

*Reforming Health Care on the Front Line
in the United States and the United Kingdom*

REBECCA KOLINS GIVAN

ILR PRESS

AN IMPRINT OF
CORNELL UNIVERSITY PRESS
ITHACA AND LONDON

First published 2016 by Cornell University Press

Printed in the United States of America

Library of Congress Cataloging-in-Publication Data

Names: Givan, Rebecca Kolins, 1975– author.
Title: Reforming health care on the front line in the United States and the
    United Kingdom / Rebecca Kolins Givan.
Other titles: Culture and politics of health care work.
Description: Ithaca : ILR Press, an imprint of Cornell University Press,
    2016. | Series: Culture and politics of health care work |
    Includes bibliographical references and index.
Identifiers: LCCN 2016003674 |
ISBN 9780801450051 (cloth : alk. paper)
Subjects: LCSH: Health care reform—United States. | Health care
    reform—Great Britain.
Classification: LCC RA395.A3 G527 2016 | DDC 362.1/0425—dc23 LC
    record available at http://lccn.loc.gov/2016003674

Cloth printing   10 9 8 7 6 5 4 3 2 1

To my parents, with gratitude

Contents

ACKNOWLEDGMENTS

The book you hold in your hands or see on your screen has been through a long journey, with perhaps an even higher number of twists and turns than are found on the usual scholarly roller coaster. I owe an enormous number of people a debt of gratitude for their support of this project as it evolved and unfolded. I am indebted to the dozens of interviewees (many of whom remain anonymous) who took the time to talk with me and share their experiences.

Stephen Bach has been a terrific collaborator and friend. Chapter 5 is based on joint research we conducted on Private Finance Initiative hospitals, some of which was previously published (Bach and Givan 2010). This research was originally conducted under the auspices of the Future of Unions in Modern Britain program at the London School of Economics, funded by the Leverhulme Trust. Colleagues in the United Kingdom, particularly at both the London School of Economics and Cardiff Business School, have provided crucial support and input at various stages of this research. Special thanks go to Rick Delbridge, Ed Heery, Sarah Jenkins, John

Kelly, Ian Kessler, David Metcalf, and Pete Turnbull. Chris Howell probably bears some responsibility for encouraging my interest in all this over two decades ago; he has been an invaluable mentor and friend. Thanks to Lena Hipp, Ruth Milkman, Ofer Sharone, Chris Tilly, and many seminar and conference participants who helped advance my thinking at some key points. The late Clete Daniel, James Gross, and David Lipsky all offered unfailing support. My thinking about employment relations in health care has been influenced and advanced by ongoing conversations with Darlene Clark, Paul Clark, Jody Hoffer Gittell, Peter Lazes, Adam Seth Litwin, and my ally and frequent collaborator, Ariel Avgar. Monica Bielski Boris remains a dear friend, trusted colleague, and fellow traveler. My students have consistently kept me on my toes. I have learned an enormous amount from so many of them—I am grateful especially to Elise Blasingame, Chad Gray, Tashlin Lakhani, Kelly Pike, and Maite Tapia for helping me think and learn.

Colleagues and comrades at Rutgers University have created an unusually supportive environment. Thanks in particular go to David Feingold, Janice Fine, Tamara Lee, Mingwei Liu, Fran Ryan, Tobias Schulze-Cleven, Susan Schurman, and Paula Voos. Adrienne Eaton deserves special acknowledgment for years of quiet mentorship and support, and for providing a model of rigorous, engaged scholarship coupled with uncompromising integrity.

Suzanne Gordon pushed me to think longer, harder, and most importantly bigger as I worked on this book. Holly Bailey is a brilliant and perceptive editor. Fran Benson waited patiently for this book and offered wise counsel along the way. Susan Bloom and Michael Bosia have been in on this project (and many others) since it was something quite different. They never fail to provide an editorial eye or a sympathetic ear, and I am so grateful to each of them. Steven Obranovich is a compassionate friend, and a gifted chef, and I'm lucky to know him.

Many colleagues have become friends without whom things would be much less lively. Thanks are insufficient for the support and good times provided by Rachel Ashworth, Richard Belfield, Jo Blanden, Teresa Casey, Chris Crowe, and Olivier Marie. Daphne Jayasinghe and Alison McDowell are key members of the Massive. The Donaldson family, the Jayacrowe family, and Catherine Lock, have opened their homes to me on my frequent research trips to the United Kingdom. The Wallace family has also housed me on research trips and on the many occasions when I just needed to re-charge. Yael Kropsky and Milena Robcis provided diversions when (and where) they were most needed. Cary Howie offered a constant supply of good humor, while navigating roadblocks, U-turns, and more.

There are so many other people who have given help in seeing this book to completion—mostly in knowing when I wanted to talk about it and when I did not. These indispensable friends include Emily Franzosa (and the 11 a.m. writing group); David Berman, Howard Yaruss, and the NYC Exploration Society; Michael Maccaferri, who is always on and always on fire; Stef Adams, Ellen Baxt, Margaret Ewing, David Geraghty, Ivan Ger-aghty, Jacob Greenberg, Amy Holmes, Nate Horrell, Matthew Hunter, Jen Izak, Heather Johnson, Daphne Kouretas, Pam Lowy, Stephanie Luce, Krissy Mahan, Katie McCall, Tom Medvetz, the Nyzito family, the Olney family, Masha Raskolnikov, Mark Rimbach, Maggie Russell-Ciardi, Ary Shalizi, FaTai Shieh, Noemi Sicherman, Sarah Soule, and Rhiannon Welch.

My family has been with me throughout, reminding me of what really matters. I thank Ben Givan, and most of all I thank my parents. This book is dedicated to them.

ABBREVIATIONS

AARP	American Association of Retired Persons
ACA	Affordable Care Act of 2010
ACAS	Advisory, Conciliation and Arbitration Service
ACO	Accountable Care Organization
ACS	American College of Surgeons
AFC	Agenda for Change
AFL-CIO	American Federation of Labor-Congress of Industrial Organizations
AHA	American Hospital Association
ANA	American Nurses' Association
BMA	British Medical Association
CMS	Centers for Medicare and Medicaid Services
CNA	California Nurses Association
GAO	US Government Accountability Office
GP	General Practitioner
HIV	Human immunodeficiency virus

HMO	Health maintenance organization
JCAH	Joint Commission for the Accreditation of Hospitals
JCAHO	Joint Commission on Accreditation of Healthcare Organizations (now the Joint Commission)
MP	Member of Parliament
NHS	National Health Service
OSHA	Occupational Safety and Health Administration
PFI	Private Finance Initiative
PPO	Preferred Provider Organization
RCN	Royal College of Nursing
SEIU	Service Employees International Union
TUPE	Transfer of Undertakings (Protection of Employment) Regulations
UAN	United American Nurses
VA	Veterans Administration
WHO	World Health Organization

THE CHALLENGE TO CHANGE

INTRODUCTION

On the eightieth anniversary of the British National Health Service (NHS), US physician Don Berwick, an unabashed fan, gave a speech expressing his great love for the NHS. "There comes a time, and the time has come," he said, "for stability, on the basis of which, paradoxically, productive change becomes easier and faster, as the good, smart, committed people of the NHS—the one million wonderful people who can carry you into the future—find the confidence to try improvements without fearing the next earthquake" (Berwick 2008). In the same speech Berwick lamented the US health care system, which he characterized as a "duplicative, supply-driven, fragmented care system" (Berwick 2008). This book examines the tension between productive improvements and unproductive "earthquakes" in both the United States and the United Kingdom. This tension is, indeed, the core problem for anyone hoping to improve health care quality anywhere.

For over a decade I have listened intently as workers and managers have described the myriad new initiatives pouring down upon them, constantly interrupting their ability to provide high quality and appropriate health care.

Policymakers routinely believe they have found a panacea—a single change that will dramatically improve health care outcomes, lower costs, or even do both. As one frustrated hospital manager told me when I asked if he was adequately consulted over new initiatives, "they do consult us; it's not clear whether they ever listen to the answers" (personal interview, March 28, 2002). This sentiment was echoed by scores of frontline workers and their managers over my years of research in hospitals in two countries, demonstrating the true challenge of implementing worthwhile change in hospitals.

In the United States and United Kingdom, health care workers, tiring of constant attempts to improve efficiency or measure performance, are complaining about their great weariness with change, sometimes known as change fatigue. In this book I examine how health care change has been implemented in hospitals in these two countries and historically what factors have combined to make meaningful, lasting change. Hospitals are the site of the preponderance of health care delivery (whether measured in patient acuity, employment, or expenditures), and they are also the most complex, sophisticated organizations in the health care sector.

Health care payers, regulatory bodies, and policymakers send initiative after initiative into the workplace, where frontline staff struggle with the constant dilemma of how to care for their patients while simultaneously pursuing initiatives that have come from outside their organizations. The push from policymakers, executives, and insurers for transformation, change, and reform in health care delivery is incessant (Berwick 2008). Private organizations, politicians, and regulators continue to push to improve performance, reduce waste, and spread best practices in hospitals. Health care providers are being encouraged or required by payers and regulators to do more with less. To comply with the onslaught of new rules and regulations, providers are expected to implement massive new information technology systems that will digitize service delivery and medical records, reduce medical errors, and make health care more patient-centered. At the same time, hospitals on both sides of the Atlantic have been required to measure everything they do and to demonstrate their high level of performance (Bevan and Hood 2006; Chassin et al. 2010).

Although health care leaders and managers around the world have been constantly preoccupied with productivity and performance, they also have a newer concern. Between 1999 and 2000, influential reports in both the United States and the United Kingdom highlighted the startling cost in human life as well as money of medical errors (Department of Health 2000, 2001; Gaffney et al. 1999; Kohn, Corrigan, and Donaldson 2000). In the United States, for example, an influential Institute of Medicine report estimated that 98,000 deaths were caused by medical errors each year, but more recent estimates suggest the figure may be as high as 400,000 deaths per year (James 2013; Kohn, Corrigan, and Donaldson 2000). Groups such as the Institute for Health Care Improvement in the United States and the National Patient Safety Agency in the United Kingdom, among many others, began to push for patient safety around the year 2000. Recent research suggests that the problem is still quite serious and that morbidity and mortality resulting from medical errors may be at far higher levels than even the earlier, attention-getting estimates (James 2013). Most of the patient-safety initiatives have been accompanied by the introduction of new technologies such as electronic medical records. Thus, payers and policymakers ask managers and frontline staff to master new computer systems, which may have their own pitfalls and introduce threats to patient safety (Koppel et al. 2005). Hospital workers and managers have therefore had to contend with yet another series of change initiatives and scoring mandates, with an attendant set of penalties for noncompliance.

Numerous public and private organizations, including the Institute for Healthcare Improvement and the Joint Commission in the United States, and the National Institute for Clinical Excellence and Dr. Foster Intelligence (an independent, university-based research body), have launched dozens of programs spotlighting the need for everything from hand-washing to team communication. Many of these vaunted programs, such as the Six Sigma Black Belt, engage only the top managers and lead physicians in a hospital and leave the key issue of staff engagement to chance (Dunn 2014). Managers and staff are somehow expected to incorporate these new initiatives into their practices while also dealing with a labor shortage in most of the skilled professions and higher demands from an aging population and improved medical technologies.

From metric-driven performance monitoring to the patient-safety movement, the only constant is change. Civil servants, researchers, and consultants craft and bring into the hospitals a cascade of change and reform initiatives with no clear rationale, and they ask managers, professionals, and other workers to accept and implement these new ideas. These initiatives often rely on highly paid external consultants to implement programs such as lean production, Six Sigma, and Hardwiring Excellence to reengineer work processes, frequently from the top down, relying on approaches imposed by outsiders without frontline experience (Vest and Gamm 2009). In spite of change fatigue and skepticism from workers about the results of initiatives that have been launched only to fail, managers and professionals seemingly face no choice but to accept, adopt, implement, and adapt these initiatives.

Enormous amounts of time, money, and energy are devoted to this process of implementation, adaptation, and acceptance. Hospital managers and staff are frequently held accountable for the successful implementation of these initiatives. At the top of the health care hierarchy, policymakers and consultants make sweeping promises about the benefits of their change initiatives. As they throw around concepts such as streamlining, efficiency, quality, and excellence, they have created a whole new health care jargon equipped with "pillars" and "belts" and lean production processes. They argue that these will produce better health outcomes at lower cost and will provide patient-centered care with greater patient satisfaction. Frontline staff—whether management, professionals, or support staff—seem to have little choice but to acquiesce to these initiatives. But they often find it difficult to initiate their own changes.

Critical Questions

What are the results of all these promises, time, and money? Do big ideas from outside the hospitals improve health care outcomes? Is change best when it is imposed from above? Does the relentless quest for change produce better patient care, greater efficiencies in health care, quality services, or even dramatic cost savings? If not, what are the results of these initiatives? When do they prompt acceptance and when do they provoke resistance? How do the organization of the workplace and its complex relationships influence the acceptance of change imposed from the outside? When and how do managers and professionals try to shape these programs to suit their own and their patients' needs? Do they succeed? Or is what results a constant series of compromises and adaptations to adaptations? When does change move from the macro to the micro, and when is the opposite true?

Over the past two decades, my work has been devoted to the health care systems in both the United States and the United Kingdom. As a long-term resident at various times and a citizen of both countries, I have become a keen observer and analyst of the evolving health care system in each. In this book I try to answer the critical questions I have just posed by examining a series of change initiatives as they are experienced at the front line in what appear to be two entirely dissimilar health care systems—the largely privatized system in the United States and the highly "socialized" (publicly funded and publicly provided) system in the United Kingdom. Using concrete examples of organizational and even systemwide change in these case studies, I investigate what happens when change is initiated both from above and from below.

I have found that wherever its point of departure in the complexities of the contemporary hospital, successful organizational change requires a deep level of acceptance and commitment not only from managers but also from staff on the front line. Indeed, some of the most successful health care change initiatives have been launched at the frontline level where workers responded to serious problems they had identified and struggled to remedy them, not only in their institutions but at the national or state level. Thus, I challenge the widely accepted notion that successful change is launched from above and trickles down with my analysis of how change also trickles *up* when frontline staff launch initiatives that eventually affect national policy.

A huge proportion of the research on health care change focuses on change initiatives that are launched by elite players such as CEOs, hospital administrators, or physician pioneers, and it neglects the possibility that change can also move up from the front line (Berry and Seltman 2008; Lee 2004). The general literature on management and health care change management has devoted an enormous amount of attention to those who make sweeping promises that the latest new initiative will prove a panacea that provides both quality and efficiency without a downside. The focus is on visionary leaders and their heroic and ultimately successful struggles to transform the corporation or hospital from top down (Berwick 1996, 2003; Pronovost et al. 2006). In this literature, workers—whether physicians or janitorial staff—are depicted as being afraid of change and as obstacles whose irrational resistance to change must be overcome.

In this book, however, I offer a more nuanced account. I examine the dual dynamic of health care delivery change in detail and with balance. I show

how high-level initiatives may indeed be distorted or subverted in hospitals, but I also explore why change is often resisted at the frontline level—sometimes with good reason—and try to help readers understand which top-down changes are resisted and why, and which are accepted, adopted, and sometimes constructively adapted and why.

While I analyze worker resistance to top-down change initiatives, I look beyond this to focus as well on a dynamic that has received very little attention: how changes initiated by frontline staff may trickle up to become policy at the macro level. These policies have produced positive changes that in turn have had significant impacts on safety, performance, and productivity. I argue that nonimplementation of a policy by frontline staff, such as occurred in the subversion of performance indicators in the United Kingdom, can shape future policy in surprising ways (see chapter 3). I also show how change can be initiated by workers while they are addressing problems that management seems to ignore and are struggling to transform the workplace in ways that make health care and the hospital safer for both patients and those who care for them. This crucial work is explored in chapter 6, which examines staff-driven initiatives to create a safety culture in hospitals that benefits both patients and employees.

Where unions are present, they play a key role in the implementation or obstruction of workplace change as well as influencing the development of policies at the national level. Key contributions of the health care unions cannot be ignored. In the United Kingdom, NHS hospitals are unionized, with a number of unions representing different occupational and professional groups; in the United States, union membership varies considerably by workplace and region across the health care industry (Milkman and Luce 2014). Although many politicians view unions as obstructionist, clinging to rigid contract language, and unwilling to embrace change, the reality is quite different. Health care unions play key roles in ensuring high-quality patient care, from facilitating ongoing communication to drawing attention to immediate problems such as poor infection control and unmet patient needs. In fact, well-run local unions with talented stewards frequently initiate change that may improve performance for everyone in the hospital—patients, staff, and management alike. As the organized voice of frontline health care workers, unions are well-positioned to identify problems and to suggest solutions in the delivery of care.

I do not presume that the role of unions is monolithic. Instead, my analysis starts from the observation that unions organize the voice of their members, and in this role they may be either proponents of or impediments to change. I examine the specific work of unions where they are present (almost everywhere in the UK health economy, and only in concentrated pockets in the United States). The chapters ahead highlight several cases in which unions have facilitated positive change, and they demonstrate that the view of unions as obstacles to change is at best antiquated and is more likely simply motivated by ideology rather than experience.

Contrasts and Commonalities

In a letter to *The Guardian* in May 2015, at a time when the NHS was a key issue in the imminent election, a group of dozens of American doctors urged the British public to proceed with caution. They affirm how much the providers in these two systems look to each other:

> There are many things the US healthcare system has to admire, such as our pioneering integrated care organizations and our world-leading medical research and high-tech rescue care. At the same time, the US is in the midst of a major healthcare reform effort that aims to bring affordability and equity to American healthcare. We caution the UK against moving in the direction of a system that has created the inequality in US that we are now working to repair. Your universal, public healthcare system is an example to the world, and something of which Britain should be proud. We urge you to preserve it. (Wang 2015)

These two countries with a common language, a common model of health care provision, and a dramatically different model of health care financing have long held an interest in each other. As both these systems contemplated changes over the last several decades, their mutual awareness of each other became evident. As privatization debates continued in the United Kingdom, observers sought evidence from the private US health care system. On the occasions that single-payer health care was discussed in recent decades in the United States, the key exemplar tended to be the United Kingdom (Light 2003). Articles with titles such as "What Are the Lessons from the USA for Clinical Commissioning Groups in the English National Health Service?" (Ham and Zollinger-Read 2012) and "A healthy debate? The US and English Health Systems" (Thorlby 2009) cropped up across the top medical, health policy, and even news publications in the United Kingdom. When private companies were given the opportunity to bid on NHS contracts, many US-based providers saw a key opportunity for profit. When a crisis of poor-quality care and high mortality rates hit the Mid-Staffordshire health care system, the US physician Don Berwick was brought in to investigate the mess. In his letter accompanying his report to senior NHS executives and government officials, he wrote, "You are stewards of a globally important treasure: the NHS" (Berwick 2013, Annex B).

This mutual awareness has often been colored by mutual suspicion. When Simon Stevens, a Brit who had spent almost a decade working in the United States as a top executive for UnitedHealth, was appointed the chief executive of NHS England in 2013, UNISON, the major public service union, responded by saying, "We sincerely hope this is not a sign that the government wants to import America-type values into the NHS and look at ways of developing healthcare through an insurance model" (UNISON 2013). Indeed, through my ongoing research on change in the two systems, I have discovered firsthand how each system looks to the other, and I have heard countless interviewees express interest, fascination, and horror in the other country's health system.

In comparisons of health systems in developed countries, the UK and US systems frequently fall at opposite poles. For example, in the Commonwealth Fund's periodic international comparison of eleven developed countries' health care systems, the United Kingdom ranks first in eight categories as well as in overall ranking whereas the United States ranks last in four categories and dead last in overall ranking (Davis et al. 2014).

Likewise, in terms of access to and payment for medical services, the US and British health care systems probably differ the most of any two in the industrialized world. The British NHS is a massive, fairly centralized single-payer, single-provider health care system. It is financed through taxation, health care providers are public employees, and access to health care is universal. In the United States, the payers and providers are far more diverse. Although the government purchases health care for more than 100 million people (including those eligible for public programs as well as public employees), most health care is purchased by employers, with a small proportion purchased by private individuals. Before the Affordable Care Act (ACA) of 2010, this fragmented system left about 50 million people without any access to health care except in the case of emergency, a far cry from the universal coverage of the NHS.

In terms of payment, the systems differ not only in who pays for health care but in how the payment systems operate. In the United States, the payment systems create massive profits for many of the stakeholders and also provide a system of incentives that do not necessarily align with the goals of providing widespread, high-quality, and efficient health care. The NHS has relatively simple payment systems in which most providers receive salaries and the system uses its large-scale purchasing power to negotiate prices on drugs, devices, and diagnostic equipment. The story is quite different in the United States, where the system is rife with incentives to treat more: doctors and hospitals profit by providing more treatment, regardless of the quality of care or the outcomes (Brownlee 2008). Physician and health care innovator Don Berwick has referred to the US system as "supply-driven care" (Berwick 2008). This is the opposite of the UK system, which is able to focus on a broad public health strategy, prevention, and a long-term outlook.

In spite of these differences, when one looks beyond access and payment into the health care workplaces, there are striking similarities. In hospitals in both countries, work organization is structured around strong, historically entrenched professional boundaries. The often-fraught relationship between nurses and doctors is almost perfectly mirrored by hospitals in both countries. Health care providers are subject to similar challenges, such as ever-changing treatment protocols, advances in technology, and the health care needs of an aging population. Both systems face shortages of professionals, and they rely on recruiting workers from abroad. Trends in patient care, such as the patient-safety movement, penetrate both systems, generating particular pressures on the health care providers. The US system may appear to be fragmented in terms of access and payment, but the role of putatively voluntary regulators, especially the Joint Commission, means that no hospital is immune from centrally determined requirements that range from specific treatment protocols to cleanliness standards.

In this book I address another characteristic shared by the two systems: both are subject to concerted pressure to change, and their experiences with change initiatives have telling similarities.

Change as It Actually Happens on the Front Lines

To explore these US and UK experiences in detail, I use personal interviews as well as documentary research to focus on four historical cases from the past decade (Table 1): in the United Kingdom, the introduction of the star rating system and the advent of privatization; in the United States, regulation by the Joint Commission and the development of a safety culture. Two cases are examples of change imposed from above, and two cases examine change initiated at the front line. I have chosen each case because it represents a crucial moment in the development of the current health care system and also traces a key ongoing trend in the Anglo-American health care model: accountability, centralized regulation, privatization and resistance, and the turn to quality. These four forces are acting on both the UK and US health care systems, even while each system has a different starting point in its current institutional configuration.

The cases I present offer evidence about the front line that moves beyond stereotypes of health care workers as frightened of change or as obstacles that invariably halt promising initiatives in their tracks. I focus instead on feedback effects that are instrumental in shaping future attempts to reform and restructure hospitals. Health care workers on the front line play a crucial role in shaping change. It is essential for would-be reformers to understand how change actually works in these complex institutions if they are to assess accurately the chances for implementing change at either the macro or the micro level. Without this deeper understanding, the parade of new initiatives, never fully implemented, will doubtless continue but will rarely cause actual improvements in the delivery of health care.

Table 1. Case studies

Case type	United Kingdom	United States
Change from above	Star rating performance measurement *Accountability*	Joint Commission Accreditation *Central regulation*
Change from below	Response to privatization *Privatization and resistance*	Movement for a safety culture *Quality*

My research on these cases is primarily qualitative and uses a multistakeholder, vertical-slice approach; that is, I have attempted to interview representatives of all the key stakeholders at all levels, from policy to practice. I also rely on primary and secondary documents, including government publications and employer and union-produced materials, to construct accurate accounts that include the perspectives of all relevant stakeholders. My interviewees included frontline health care workers and managers, local, regional, and national union representatives, and bureaucrats and elected officials. Most of the interviews in the United Kingdom were conducted between 2002 and 2007, with a few later interviews in subsequent years. The US interviews were primarily conducted from 2007 to 2014. I summarize the interviews and offer select representative quotations. Most interviews were conducted individually, for thirty to ninety minutes, although there were a handful of group interviews (from a two-person interview to a ten-person focus group) and a small number of telephone interviews as well. The high-level interviewees, such as those from national regulators, were specifically selected for their expertise. The frontline interviewees were selected in hospitals that represented the diversity of hospital workplaces in each country.

These interviews, as well as extensive documentary research, make up the empirical data used throughout the book. These diverse perspectives illuminate the sometimes conflicting interests of the different stakeholders in health care. Although I have not interviewed patients for this study, the research is informed, where appropriate, by patient data, including surveys reflecting patient satisfaction as well as quantitative measures of clinical outcomes. Elsewhere in my research, I have given patient sources a great deal more emphasis (see, for example, Avgar, Givan, Liu 2011a, 2011b; Givan, Avgar, Liu 2010). Although there is occasionally patient-led change in the provision of health care, this is a rare occurrence compared with change initiated by frontline providers or national regulators.[1]

---

1. The best example of patient-led change is probably the change in labor and delivery practices as part of the women's movements of the 1960s and 1970s. Women wrested some control of their delivery environments from doctors, and forced doctors and hospitals to allow partners and others chosen by the birthing mother to remain in the delivery room. Expectant mothers chose hospitals that would allow them this control over their birthing environment, and this competition then drove widespread adoption of the new practice. My thanks to Ellen Berman for suggesting this example of patient-driven change in health care delivery.

Theoretical Bases

There is a rich literature in political science, sociology, and comparative political economy on welfare state institutions and welfare state reform. Health care is a pillar of any welfare state, and it is crucial to understand the constraints on and possibilities for change in health care as part of the welfare state more broadly. By including a macro level examination of these health care systems, my analysis demonstrates the relationship between national institutions and policies and the front line of service where these policies become practice.

In terms of this research tradition there are two main reasons for comparing the health care workplace in the United States and United Kingdom. First, the research is in the tradition of "most different systems" comparison and asks why, in spite of such different national institutions, the dynamic in the health care workplace is so similar in both countries (Meckstroth 1975). If one looks only at national institutions (such as the regulatory and payment systems and the role of health insurance companies), one would not expect these workplace relationships to be similar. Rather, the national institutional settings reveal massive differences in who pays for health care and who has access to health care. But in the workplaces of the two countries there are striking similarities. In particular, the relationships between professional and occupational groups, the competing needs of (and incentives for) different stakeholders, and the shortage of skilled health care professionals in the workforce (exacerbated by major retention problems) combine to create health care workplaces that bear more than a family resemblance. Health care providers in the United Kingdom and the United States have also faced similar imperatives for increased productivity and enhanced performance, as calculated using a range of sometimes controversial measures. These pressures emanate from national bodies: in the United Kingdom there is a centralized regulatory system; in the United States a series of overlapping voluntary and mandatory regulatory bodies create a kind of de facto national regulation. These similar trends in the face of systemic differences require a deeper analysis, focused at the front line of health care, the workplace.

The second reason for comparing a sector across Britain and the United States is that the economies of these two countries have been grouped together by scholars eager to create simple typologies and frameworks. The now dominant typology of varieties of capitalism classified both economies as liberal market economies, characterized by relatively light regulation and a low degree of economic coordination (Hall and Soskice 2001). Esping-Andersen's seminal study of welfare states classified both welfare states as liberal welfare regimes, with welfare functioning only as a safety net for the neediest and a general reliance on the market; the United States, however, was a much neater example of this regime than the United Kingdom (Esping-Andersen 1990). In their work on changing employment systems in industrialized countries, Katz and Darbishire (2000) found that both the British and American economies have featured declining union representation, increased inequality, and similar variations in employment and human resources practices across industries.

In studying health care workplaces, it is essential to view the process of ongoing change in context—that is, as part of a series of relationships (or institutional interactions) stemming from and feeding back to these same institutions (Pierson 1994). In other words, the government and large employers—and indeed insurance companies—create policy using a variety of considerations from workplace consultation to electoral politics. A complex configuration of interests influences the direction of policy and its ultimate success.

The NHS is a huge single-payer, single-provider public health care system, covering the entire population of about 60 million people. In contrast, the US system is a primarily private system that features a predominantly employment-based insurance system and, until the implementation of the ACA, excluded about 50 million people from access to regular health care. The ownership, insurance, and payment structures in the two countries could not be more different. In the United States, health care is both the largest and the fastest growing industry and has more than 18 million employees in almost 1.4 million workplaces (US Bureau of Labor Statistics 2015)(Bureau of Labor Statistics 2008). In the United Kingdom, about 1.2 million people are directly employed by the NHS, with more providing outsourced support services and contracted core services (Workforce and Facilities Team 2015).

The UK health care system is highly centralized, with 90 percent of the entire health care sector owned and operated by the central government. In contrast, the US system is a tangled web of payers and providers. This includes private hospitals and insurance companies as well as some government-owned and -operated programs (in particular, the Veterans Administration and the Indian Health Service) in addition to government-funded programs that are privately provided—most significantly Medicare and Medicaid. Ownership, payment, and access are the starkest differences between the US health care system and the British NHS.

In spite of major differences in the financing and ownership of these health care systems, there are important similarities. In both countries hospitals are the biggest organizations providing health care, and the government is the biggest purchaser of care. Inside the hospital workplaces in the two countries, the similarities become even more apparent. Entrenched professional roles, resistance to change, and shortages of skilled staff are key concerns in both countries.

Hospitals in both the United States and the United Kingdom face many of the same current pressures. These common pressures are elucidated in the cases in the chapters that follow. The push for increased accountability and monitoring, improved quality, centralized regulation and standardization, and the tug-of-war for and against privatization, competition, and neoliberalism are trends that can be seen across the Anglo-American systems. These forces cut across the operations of hospitals in both countries. They are the forces behind the changes that create the titular challenges of the cases described herein. These goals and objectives motivate the constant parade of changes in health care. These four categories represent the *what* of the changes, and the cases here describe the *how* of the changes—How do they start? How are they initiated and by whom? And when and why are they successful or unsuccessful?

Much of the research on health care institutions has placed health care within the broader institutions and relationships of the welfare state. Like other welfare institutions, such as education and pensions, health care straddles the public and private sectors. In the fields of political science and sociology there has been a vigorous debate among competing explanations for welfare state (including health care institutions) formation, expansion, and retrenchment. Most of these explanations focus on the entrenched interests of welfare beneficiaries rather than on providers. Many theories of the welfare state seek to explain the creation of the welfare state rather than changes in welfare state institutions (Immergut 1992; Mares 2000; Pizzorno 1978; Swenson 2002). The major theories focus on the policy aspects of the welfare state, specifically when and how major welfare legislation is created and passed (Giaimo and Manow 1999; Immergut 1992; Mares 2000; Pierson

1996; Pizzorno 1978; Swenson 2002). These scholars did not examine when, how, or whether this legislation, once passed, is implemented. Even Giaimo's examination of the implementation of health care reform analyzed only modes of health care financing, an aspect that does not explain the major changes in modes of service delivery in Britain. Her assertion that "employers and government policy makers, and their interest in cost containment have become the driving force behind welfare state reform" (2001, 334) may have been an accurate description of Britain in the Thatcher era, but it did not reflect the massive increase in health care spending in Britain or the United States in many (but not all) recent years.

The vertical-slice framework I use allows for the analysis of health care restructuring where the rubber meets the road, at the front line of health care provision. I track policy changes from the point of initiation, whether within the workplace or at the national level, to implementation at the front line of care delivery. Essential to my argument here is an understanding of policy feedback, as explicated by Paul Pierson (1994). As he argues, once welfare institutions and entitlements are entrenched in a society, the possibilities for change become constrained. He rightly shows that policies and welfare institutions create new and powerful interest groups that in turn shape future policy. This feedback effect, in its simplest form, is a demonstration of the way that past policy constrains future policy because of the role of entrenched interest groups. I contend that welfare state employees on the front line, in addition to recipients of welfare benefits on whom Pierson focuses, can shape the process and possibilities for welfare reform, particularly in the labor-intensive health care sector. The vertical slice, cutting across the whole system from the policy level to the workplace, allows us to see how policies and institutions create interest groups in the workplace, which in turn enable and constrain future policy and practice.

It is also worth noting that in the case of health care in Britain and the United States there is no retrenchment or decline. Instead, there has been a continual process of restructuring, coupled with an increase in employment and expenditure in both countries. Pierson's key examples of the process of policy feedback in the welfare state are of services and transfer payments under threat (such as housing and pension payments). In the case of health care restructuring, there is no direct organizing among service recipients. Rather, the service providers have much more to lose with the imposition of new ways of working and new governance structures in their workplaces.

Giaimo and Manow (1999) made a strong case for examining policy implementation as well as policy formation in the study of health care reform. In particular, they rebutted scholars who explained welfare policy reform by way of party politics: "We do not deny the importance of explanations focused on the political arena, but we find that they tell only part of the story of policy change. In particular, such explanations tend to focus on the legislative process and thus can only answer the question of whether a policy was enacted or not. They give only a partial explanation for why policy makers settled on the particular content of reforms and often fail to consider events within a given sector at the implementation stage" (969).

The framework I use affirms the assertion that policy implementation is crucial. Key workplace structures determine whether and how health care reform is implemented. Giaimo and Manow focus on the role of the health care payers in determining the possibilities for reform. This explanation seems somewhat apt for their US and German cases, but it cannot explain the British case in which private companies are eager to profit from health care and the key existing payer remains the state (Monbiot 2000). Payers may exert influence over the degree of marketization of health care provision, but employees can affect all forms of frontline service delivery with or without competition in both the public and private sectors.

The history of performance ratings in chapter 3 demonstrates the political effects of the policy changes envisioned by Pierson. It describes how the ratings regime brought out the interests of hospital managers, who in turn were able to eliminate the ratings policy. But while Pierson focuses on the interests of recipients of welfare benefits, I focus on the interests of welfare state employees and the workplace effects of policy changes.

Pierson has argued that interest groups create policy, and policies also create interest groups. His paradigmatic example is that of social security. According to Pierson, the US Social Security program created a group with common interests—the recipients—who then became an organized interest group—the American Association of Retired Persons (AARP). The AARP was a product of a particular policy, but it became a powerful interest group with the ability to influence future policy (Pierson 1994). In the case of health care, it is not only health care beneficiaries that have become an organized interest group but also health care providers. Although some scholars have shown the importance of physicians in the establishment of health care systems (Immergut 1992; Starr 1982), the creation of new interest groups, with the exception of patient advocacy groups, and their ability to shape future policy has been largely ignored. This is particularly true of all nonphysician health care providers. The traditional professional status hierarchy is reinforced by scholars of health care change who, in many cases, foreground the role of physicians (and sometimes executives) while diminishing the essential roles of other staff groups.

There is a powerful feedback effect through which current health care institutions shape—or even create—interest groups, which in turn have a strong influence over the possibilities for future change and the production of future policy. It is not possible to understand this feedback effect by looking only at the policymaking level or only at the national level. Rather, much of the action that determines the future of both health care delivery and policy happens at the workplace, where managers and frontline staff are charged with implementing the barrage of new initiatives. The example of star ratings in the British NHS (set out in chapter 3) demonstrates how the distorted implementation of a policy at the workplace led to the abandonment of this policy.

Although change imposed from above can be problematic, there are exciting innovations trickling up from the front line. When they are present, unions are a key facilitator of feedback, although they are not the only outlet for frontline staff voice. The frontline professionals and staff who have the most direct and intimate knowledge of the challenges of their work frequently come up with initiatives that improve health care for everyone. At times, the initiatives can move from a single workplace to become the norm (whether through regulation or the dissemination of best practice). The use of checklists in surgery is one such initiative, albeit physician initiated rather than initiated by nurses or other health care staff (Berenholtz et al. 2004; Gawande 2009a; Pronovost et al. 2006), the mandatory use of safety needles to prevent needle-stick injuries (discussed in chapter 6) is another. These cases demonstrate the power of frontline workers' knowledge, which cannot be replicated by someone outside the organization. It is worth noting, however, that those programs created and promoted by physicians tend to achieve much quicker traction than those initiated by nurses, other health care professionals, or indeed lower status, lower paid staff in hospitals.

One of the primary tensions in hospitals is between managers and professionals. Professions have developed over centuries, with strong identities, professional autonomy, and respect for specific knowledge and skills (for much more on the history of nursing and medicine, see Nelson 2001; Starr 1982). Traditionally, professionals have controlled entry to their own profession by controlling the licensure or credentialing process. In health care, nursing and medicine are the largest professions, but there are scores of other essential professionals such as pharmacists and social workers. Through the evolution of health care institutions in both countries, the role of nonprofessional managers has grown dramatically. Most hospitals now have a chief medical officer, a chief nursing officer, and a chief executive officer (although there is wide variation in actual job titles).

The chief executive is the final arbiter and theoretically sits above the top physician and nurse managers in the organizational hierarchy. In practice, however, it is almost impossible for a nonphysician to impose anything on the physicians against their will. Enter any hospital in the United Kingdom or the United States, and one encounters the constant complaints of doctors refusing to cooperate or follow orders, complaints emanating from management, nurses, and other staff. The professionals in turn assert that their professional authority trumps any suggestions or recommendation from nonprofessionals. This major tension exists in hospitals in both the United Kingdom and the United States and certainly transcends the structural and financial differences in the two health care systems. The relationship between management and professionals has the potential to strain implementation of any reform initiatives. For an initiative to succeed, all frontline staff generally have to agree on and support the process as well as the overarching objectives—lack of buy-in from professionals makes it impossible for management to make any changes.

The Challenge to Change Now

The questions of the causes of and obstacles to successful changes to improve health care are more relevant now than ever. As health care workers face this flood of change initiatives, policymakers, health care researchers, administrators, and elite physicians are proposing one initiative after another to make health care safer, more rational, or more satisfying to patients. In the United States, the most sweeping health care legislation in decades promises to reshape access to and payment for health care without having much effect on the health care workplace. The 2010 ACA mainly creates incremental change in the health insurance market, but policymakers and consultants, insurance companies and professionals are clamoring to take advantage of the opportunity to shape broader changes.

In the United Kingdom under Tony Blair's Labor government, the push was not to do more with less, but to do even more with more. Expenditure and employment increased, but so did the number of change initiatives. From performance monitoring to annual surveys of staff and patients, from the gradually increasing role of the private sector to the growth in use of nonprofessional staff (especially health care assistants), new initiatives and new pressures became the norm. The onslaught of change initiatives has continued, even as the coalition and then Conservative governments of David Cameron implemented austerity measures that choked off health service funding.

The British NHS is the most centralized and socialized health care system, while the United States system is the most fragmented and relies on private insurance and private provision of care. The differences in these systems are in access and payment, not in the delivery of care at the front line. In fact, hospitals in both countries bear striking similarities. As the following chapters elaborate, frontline workers in both countries face many of the same challenges, from interprofessional collaboration to infection control. While the British system is explicitly nationally regulated, the regulatory framework in the American system is less well known. Nevertheless, the scale of government-purchased health care and the scope of national regulation mean that hospitals in the United States are underpinned by a common set of rules of operation. Although payment systems in the United States are fragmented and access to health care is not universal, American hospitals are subject to uniform rules and pressures that have much in common with their counterparts in the United Kingdom.

Many in the United Kingdom see the US health care system as their worst nightmare: "Thank God for the NHS. Thank God the NHS didn't go the American way," said one general practitioner after seeing Michael Moore's film *Sicko* (Edemariam, Henley, and Khaleeli 2007). In the United States, the fear of socialized medicine was ever present in the 2009–10 health care reform debate, and ultimately the fear of stifling free markets led to the demise of a public health care option. In a laughable moment at the height of the health care debate in the United States, former New York City mayor Rudolph Giuliani alleged, with blatant disregard for the facts, that if he had had prostate cancer in the United Kingdom rather than the United States, he would be dead. Yet as employees and patients of each system fear their idea of the other, the systems are moving gradually closer together, with an increase in government-purchased health care in the United States after the Medicaid expansion in the ACA, and a growing role for private providers contracted to the NHS in the United Kingdom.

While I focus of the difficulty of implementing change in both systems, my analysis secondarily sheds light on some of the essential similarities between hospitals in both countries. There is no better way to examine the dynamic between change at the micro and the macro levels than by looking at the two health care systems in the industrialized world that seem the most diametrically opposed: the United States and the United Kingdom. The primary research is contextualized with historical accounts of key moments of change in each system. The argument and the data presented in this book reveal that workers and managers in systems thought to be so dissimilar respond to change initiatives in similar ways. This insight helps us to understand the processes that influence system change and creates a much clearer picture of the importance of the front line in any potential systemic change. Exploring these similarities, I trace change initiatives imposed from above and those initiated at the workplace level. In the process, I demonstrate that many of the most significant and successful change initiatives in both countries have moved not from the macro level to the micro but from the micro to the macro.

My analysis of the two health care systems frames a key argument: not only do national institutions shape workplace relationships, but workplace relationships can also shape national institutions. Among the examples detailed in the chapters that follow are the workplace response to the Private Finance Initiative in the United Kingdom, which led to new regulations restricting the ability of private contractors to degrade the pay and conditions of privatized workers. Similarly, both the use of safety needles and the widespread adoption of checklists to eliminate errors and infections, practices that were initiated by frontline staff in US hospitals, have now become embedded in national regulations. In these cases of bottom-up change, we see that the configuration of national institutions does not determine the outcome in the workplace. Rather, the workplace relationships and the ability of employees to solve pressing problems by applying their own expertise and then propagating successful initiatives more broadly have reshaped national practice.

This argument stands in stark contrast to much of the established literature on employment relations. The received wisdom in political economy and industrial relations, as argued in numerous seminal books (including volumes by Hall and Soskice 2001; Katz and Darbishire 2000; Kochan, Katz, and McKersie 1986; Piore and Sabel 1984) is that national institutions shape workplace relationships. The influence of workplace relationships on national institutions, however, has been largely overlooked. Nevertheless, as I show in the chapters that follow, the experiences of workers on the front line can and do shape future policy.

Whether and how policy is both made and implemented is profoundly affected by what is happening in the workplace. Legislators and regulators cannot simply create change by writing it into the law. Rather, the messy reality of the workplace may distort, pervert, accelerate, or enhance the intended policy. Similarly, national change may begin in the workplace when frontline workers are most aware of the causes of problems and the likely areas for improvement. When local initiatives from frontline workers are successful, the policy diffuses and sometimes moves from a practice that is voluntary or covered in a collective bargaining agreement to a law covering all workplaces, regardless of employer or employee preferences or union coverage.

This book focuses directly on the relationship between national policy and workplace practice and the feedback dynamic that determines this relationship. National policy and institutions structure workplace relationships, which in turn have an impact on future policies and institutional changes. Too often one side of this two-way relationship has been overemphasized to the neglect of the other.

Overview of the Chapters Ahead

To make a convincing case for a dynamic found across two countries and at the intersection of policy and practice, it is necessary to take a deep dive into each country's health care system before moving to the more contemporary cases. In chapters 1 and 2, I provide a history of each country's health care system with an introduction to the key stakeholders and an explanation of how and why they came to hold their current positions. These are not comprehensive histories but rather long looks at the ongoing processes of change that have led to the current institutional configuration.

I contextualize the long history of change in health care in both countries and make detailed comparisons of the unending attempts at change in hospitals in both the United Kingdom and the United States. I introduce the key players in each system—the payers, providers, and patients—and explain how each system has evolved into its current form. In the case of the United Kingdom, the NHS hospitals were relatively constant from the service's founding in 1948 until the mid-1980s. Since the 1980s, change initiatives have proliferated, from the use of outsourcing to the emphasis on performance monitoring and restructured pay systems. NHS managers and staff alike are frustrated by the constant attempts at change imposed from above, often with little consultation of the frontline staff who will be responsible for implementation.

In the United States the fragmented health care system has seen nonstop changes for at least the last half century. With the introduction of Medicaid and Medicare requirements, hospitals reoriented their delivery systems; with the introduction and legislative encouragement of health maintenance organizations (HMOs), the systems were reoriented again. The role of the Joint Commission (formerly the Joint Commission on Accreditation of Healthcare Organizations, or JCAHO) is constantly evolving. The Joint Commission is the de facto national regulator of hospitals, so when the commission establishes a new requirement (as it does regularly), frontline staff are forced to respond to its directives. The initial chapters of this book illustrate that the current, sometimes fraught, relationship between national actors and frontline health care providers is determined by long-standing interests and is not a new phenomenon. They also show that both health care systems have experienced constant change, with very little time for a new equilibrium to ever take hold.

After the introduction of the two health care systems and the key stakeholders therein, I move in the subsequent chapters to crucial case studies. These cases trace the process of implementing change and look for the sources of success and failure in that process. Chapter 3 presents an in-depth case history that relates what is ultimately an episode of failed change from above. At the turn of the twenty-first century, the British government decided to impose a star rating system on British hospitals. This new system heralded a regime of reward and punishment that has been remarkably persistent, in spite of the fact that most frontline providers find it to be detrimental to the delivery of high-quality health care. An early example of the programs of accountability and performance measurement that have become central across the US and British health care systems, the star rating system was designed to reward good performance, punish poor performance, and enable easy comparisons. At the hospital level, however, the star rating system was manipulated, and managers had no confidence in the system. I present detailed evidence from my research in hospitals that received good ratings and those that received bad ratings that reveals that the system suffered from very low credibility and it never had the buy-in of the managers who were supposed to both implement and learn from the rating system. As a result, the managers, who resented the burden of data collection and did not feel motivated by the incentives that were supposedly inherent in the system, subverted the system. The ratings process was eventually abandoned (or at least adapted beyond recognition) in response to the deep subversion of the implementation process. The case of these performance ratings illustrates the power of frontline workers to embrace, reject, or indeed subvert national policy. The ultimate abandonment of this performance rating regime is a perfect example of the feedback effect, where the workplace relationships in turn affect national policy.

The example of change from above in the United States focuses on national regulation. The regulatory entity used in the United States is the Joint Commission (formerly known as JCAHO), which is officially voluntary but plays, as Chapter 4 details, the de facto role of a mandatory credentialing agency. Health insurance companies and government reimbursement programs have essentially ceded control of hospital accreditation to the Joint Commission, so the commission acts as a de facto national regulator, imposing uniform rules and standards on hospitals across the country. I analyze the central role of the Joint Commission in imposing new initiatives on US hospitals. Every time the Joint Commission introduces a new goal, hospital staff have little choice but to comply with it, almost regardless of any adverse effects. Chapter 4 analyzes the imposition and implementation of the Joint Commission requirements as a case of an ongoing attempt at change from above leading to intense frustration and change fatigue on the front line. Criticism of these requirements from frontline staff has ultimately led to a dismissive approach to the accreditation process, such that it is seen as a wasteful bureaucratic exercise rather than an important check on patient care protocols. This is not so much a case of absolute failure but of major pushback at the point of implementation, after frontline workers have had a chance to wrestle with the impracticalities of the new rules and procedures.

In chapter 5 I show how the feedback loop works in practice. This case demonstrates pushback from the front line. Focusing on the United Kingdom, chapter 5 details the work of unions (especially UNISON) to build strong local organizations to fight the creeping privatization of the NHS. This chapter is based on research conducted jointly over several years with Stephen Bach, some of which has been published elsewhere (Bach and Givan 2010; Givan and Bach 2007). It was not a case of new policies initiated in the workplace but rather a case of feedback—workers and their unions were profoundly unhappy with the inequities that came with private sector involvement in the NHS, and they were ultimately able to force the government to protect the pay and conditions of their members. The union did fight the policy of privatization nationally (especially the Private Finance Initiative), but its most influential efforts took place in the workplace. Outsourced workers fought for better working conditions in their own hospitals while giving their national union the information and resources necessary ultimately to end the so-called two-tier workforce (the system in which workers doing the same job were paid differently depending on whether they had been employed by a public or private employer). In chapter 5 I show that change from above may beget change from below, and I demonstrate the feedback effect in action. The Private Finance Initiative created hospitals where staff worked under both public and private employers, with different terms, conditions, and benefits. The staff were able to organize themselves and respond with new initiatives, and ultimately they achieved a more equitable outcome.

In the next example of change initiated in the workplace I look at responses to the crisis in hospital safety for both patients and hospital staff. Although there have been problems with hospital safety for decades, a confluence of interests had made it difficult to legislate an improved safety culture in hospitals. In chapter 6, I provide an analysis of key safety initiatives, pushed by nurses and doctors, that have made hospitals safer places for all who set foot in them, employees or patients. I demonstrate how one nurse in one workplace took a stand that led to a national change. Lorraine Thiebaud was a nurse in San Francisco from the early days of the acquired immunodeficiency syndrome (AIDS) epidemic. After her coworker was infected with the human immunodeficiency virus (HIV) through a dangerous needle, Thiebaud took action. From the grievance procedure to a new collective bargaining agreement, and from a new state law to a new federal law, Thiebaud fought to mandate that employers purchase only safer (but more expensive) needles to protect the health and safety of their workers.

In my discussion I emphasize the importance of a multistakeholder perspective. Needle-stick injuries to staff may have only an indirect impact on patient care, but the sustainability of the workforce and the need to maintain adequate health and safety standards cannot be separated from high-quality patient care. A nurse working in an unsafe environment cannot provide the highest level of care to a patient. In this case, a nurse (and her union) recognized this and initiated a change that trickled up to the very highest level, federal legislation. I also discuss how surgical staff found a way to enforce hand-washing protocols and significantly reduce the incidence of potentially fatal central-line infections. The examples in chapter 6 demonstrate the process through which a nurse or doctor recognized a problem, developed a solution, and confronted the institutional barriers to implementing the solution. Through a gradual process, these frontline staff initiated policies that affect all US health care workers and patients.

In the conclusion, chapter 7, I draw findings from the in-depth case studies and reaffirm the feedback dynamic among legislation, regulation, and the workplace. My discussion moves from the workplace to the level of national institutions and national health care systems and revisits the relationship between workers on the front line and the implementation of national change. I show the ways in which health care providers are a critical interest group with the ability to veto, constrain, and undo attempts to change health care delivery. I elaborate on the relationship between the micro and macro levels and draw comparisons between the United Kingdom and the United States. This elucidates the claim that the US and UK health care systems are radically different in terms of payment and access but remarkably similar at the workplace level—for example, in their similar relationships between doctors and nurses. I emphasize the relationship between national health care institutions and the front line of health care delivery. As I return to the macro level, I make clear that it is not possible to understand the potential for systemic change in health care without understanding the dynamics of change at the site of most health care delivery, the hospital workplace.

Chapter 1

HEALTH CARE SYSTEMS IN THE UNITED STATES AND THE UNITED KINGDOM

A Lifetime of Change

In the United States, a woman who is delivering a baby will face different choices depending on her health insurance status. Around half of births are covered by Medicaid, the government-run health insurance program for the poor (Markus et al. 2013). Other births are covered by private health insurance, which is usually employer-sponsored but may also be purchased individually. In all these cases, the insurer or the state administering Medicaid benefits determines what kind of labor and delivery services are available. Home births and midwife-assisted births are not always covered. Depending on the insurance plan, the expectant mother may or may not have had a choice of hospitals and doctors. Insurers also vary widely in the length of hospital stay they will cover. Although expectant mothers do have some choices, they are constrained by the insurer rather than by the professional discretion of doctors and midwives. After a birth, families will receive a bill for the costs not covered by their insurance (co-pays and deductibles for both mother and infant). For those with insurance, out-of-pocket costs for childbirth (excluding pre- and postpartum care) average more than $3,000 (Rosenthal 2013).

When a British woman is pregnant, she meets her midwife, usually through her local family doctor. She chooses where to give birth: at home with a midwife, at a birthing center, or in a hospital, depending on her specific needs and where she is most comfortable. The expectant parents can take antenatal classes, usually at a local hospital or clinic. After the birth, the new mother is discharged when she and her doctor and midwife decide both mother and baby are ready. There are then a series of home visits, first by a midwife and then a health visitor, to ensure that both the mother and infant are progressing appropriately. All of this happens without the intervention of insurance companies or billing departments. The entire pre-, intra-, and post-natal experience costs the new mother nothing, and costs the National Health Service an average of under £3,000 (around US $4,500) per delivery.

The contrasts between the organizational and financial structures of the health care systems in the United States and the United Kingdom could not be stronger. Yet the pressure that change initiatives bring to bear on both systems affects them similarly. This chapter contextualizes each country's health care system and illustrates their ongoing evolution through constant attempts to change. It is crucial to understand the structure of each health care system to understand how and when change works.

How the Systems Work

In the United States

In the United States, about 18.5 million people work in the health care sector (US Bureau of Labor Statistics 2015). Of these, about 4 million are registered nurses (RNs), and around 900,000 are physicians (Henry J. Kaiser Family Foundation 2015b). Although the US health care infrastructure is ostensibly privately controlled, it is not a truly private system. In fact, the government has its tentacles in almost every aspect of health care. Although exact numbers are hard to pin down, the government purchases health insurance for about 110 million Americans, including public employees, active military and veterans, and Medicare and Medicaid recipients (whose ranks are growing since the implementation of the 2014 provisions of the Affordable Care Act of 2010) as well as those eligible for smaller government programs such as prison health care and the Indian Health Service (Henry J. Kaiser

Family Foundation 2015a; Pew Charitable Trusts, and MacArthur Foundation 2014; US Office of Personnel Management 2014). Government reimbursement programs, especially Medicare and Medicaid, determine many protocols for health care delivery. Because it is unrealistic for most hospitals to follow one set of procedures for these patients and another for privately insured patients, the government-mandated procedures often prevail for all patients. Similarly, the government (federal and state) plays a crucial regulatory role, from the US Food and Drug Administration's drug approval processes to the licensing and credentialing of health care professionals and the facilities in which they work.

The Patient Protection and Affordability Act of 2010 (commonly called the Affordable Care Act, ACA, or Obamacare) incrementally builds on the existing fragmented system of payment and service provision. The new law attempts to insure the majority of the uninsured—through Medicaid, through subsidies for purchasing private insurance, or through restricting the ability of insurers to reject patients. In this sense, the law does not dramatically change the system but rather simply expands it. The key elements of this act shift uninsured Americans into an existing form of health coverage. In most states, the income cap for Medicaid expansion was raised by the ACA, so many more people are receiving government-purchased health care; this is officially controlled by the states but with a great deal of regulatory control from both the Centers for Medicare and Medicaid Services (CMS) and the Joint Commission (as discussed later). The so-called exchanges created by the ACA also provide a mechanism for individuals to purchase health care insurance through private for-profit and not-for-profit insurers. Overall, the major provisions of Obamacare change who can access health care (especially nonemergency care) and how this care is purchased, but they do not change the provision of care or the work of health care providers on the front line.

This fragmented network of payers, including the government, insurers, and individuals, purchases the actual health care from a fragmented set of health care providers. Some organizations, such as Kaiser Permanente, function as both the insurer and the health care provider—these forms of health care insurance are often considered prepaid health care plans. The private health care providers include hospitals, clinics, and nursing homes—of which hospitals provide the most labor- and resource-intensive care. Hospitals may be either publicly owned or owned by a health care conglomerate, which may be either nonprofit or for profit. Hospitals provide health care services to patients, and the services are usually at least partially reimbursed either by a for-profit insurance company or a government program such as Medicare or Medicaid.

The ownership of US hospitals is dispersed and fragmented, but the regulation of hospitals is highly consistent and centralized. The key regulatory body is not a government agency but a voluntary, nonprofit organization, the Joint Commission (formerly the Joint Commission for the Accreditation of Health Care Organizations or JCAHO). When Medicare and Medicaid were introduced, JCAHO accreditation was the requirement for hospitals to be eligible for participation. This simple decision made it, in practice, almost mandatory for hospitals to seek accreditation—for without accreditation, the hospital would not be able to provide services to a high proportion of potential patients. The de facto unified system of regulation creates parallels with the British system, where procedures and protocols are determined by national agencies such as the National Institute for Clinical Excellence. The crucial role of the Joint Commission belies the contention that the US system is driven by market incentives or competition.

In addition to the Joint Commission, the key government agency that effectively regulates hospitals is the CMS. The CMS selects the accreditation required for health care providers to be eligible for reimbursement when providing services to Medicare or Medicaid patients. In practice, the CMS has given the Joint Commission the accrediting authority for almost every type of covered service. Although neither the Joint Commission nor the CMS are fully mandatory regulatory agencies (although many states use their standards as their accreditation standards), in practice they are universal. As such, there is national regulation of hospitals, even within the complex web of payment and ownership.

In addition to the role conferred on the Joint Commission by the CMS, many states use Joint Commission accreditation as a legal requirement for health care providers. Similarly, many health insurers will cover only services from Joint Commission–accredited providers. This means that health care providers, for all their fragmentation, are conforming to a fixed, centralized set of protocols and requirements emanating from a single entity. As one hospital administrator (a physician) put it, "I would say that by and large what is required by CMS and by the Joint Commission are the major drivers here."

This means that almost all health care facilities seek Joint Commission accreditation and conform to the standards prescribed by the Joint Commission. This is the key aspect of the de facto centralized regulation of the US health care system. These health care facilities are not owned or managed by a single entity, but this regulatory system, which is hardly voluntary, creates a single set of standards, procedures, and protocols for all health care facilities. More than 95 percent of hospital beds in the United States are in hospitals accredited by the Joint Commission (Schyve 2000).

The approximate British counterpart of the Joint Commission is the Care Quality Commission (formerly known as both the Commission for Health Care Improvement and the Health Care Commission), which monitors performance in National Health Service (NHS) facilities. Because health care provision in the United Kingdom is automatically funded by the government, the Care Quality Commission's monitoring does not make a facility eligible for payment or reimbursement but rather simply allows it to provide services. Hospitals in both countries operate within a strict system of surveillance and monitoring. In the United Kingdom the monitor is explicitly a government agency; in the United States the monitor is an independent nonprofit organization, and cooperation is nominally voluntary.

There are also various national associations that advocate for the health care industry, and their role is to lobby for their members. These organizations include America's Health Insurance Plans, whose member companies provide health insurance to more than 200 million Americans, which is the vast majority of Americans with employer-sponsored private insurance plans (America's Health Insurance Plans 2010). Similarly, most hospitals are members of the American Hospital Association (AHA), a trade group that lobbies on their behalf. The AHA describes itself as performing the functions of both a trade association and an advocate of the public interest, but many health care unions and other activists for reform have cast the AHA as rather obstructionist.

In the United Kingdom

For patients in the NHS, all care is focused around a local family doctor (the general practitioner or GP). The GPs are responsible for the overall health of their patients and take charge of most routine care and screening. They are the key point of dissemination for public health initiatives, such as smoking cessation programs. The GPs are also responsible for referring patients to specialists, and the new NHS Constitution requires that patients be given a choice of specialists and hospitals for these referrals. Since the Health and Social Care Act of 2012, GPs have also been responsible for "purchasing" the health care needed by their patients on the internal market of the NHS through the process known as commissioning.

For the typical NHS employee, the system is similarly integrated. Almost a third of NHS staff are RNs. The typical nurse works in an acute care hospital, although there are also nurses based in the community and in local family practices. Although the top executives of the hospital have a good deal of operational autonomy, the nurse's pay and terms and conditions of employment are determined nationally. Health care is nationalized, so there is no need for health insurance as part of the benefits package, and nurses receive a defined benefit pension, also determined nationally. The nurse is likely to be a member of a union, either the Royal College of Nursing or UNISON, which she joined while still a student. The nurse is managed by a nurse manager, who works in close coordination with other professional and nonprofessional members of the hospital team. For the nurse, the structure of her day-to-day work is much like that of nurses in other countries. There is a fairly strict hierarchy both among nurses and between nurses and other professionals, especially doctors.

How the Systems Came to Be

Evolution of the US System

The US health care economy has a long, complex history that has been extensively documented and analyzed elsewhere. Many historical accounts of the US health care system have focused on organized interests at the national level, such as unions and business (see Gottschalk 2000) and the medical profession (see Starr 1982). These accounts argue that the dominance of employment-based health insurance served the mutual interests of organized labor, employers, and doctors. Indeed, the combined interests of doctors, business, and labor defeated attempts to introduce compulsory health insurance early in the twentieth century (Starr 1982, 252–57). Even at this early stage in the evolution of health care institutions, however, the foundations were in place for the complex workplace relationships between professionals and other employees, and between the payers and the providers of health care.

Employment-based health insurance rose to dominance during and after World War II, following the failure of several attempts to create a national health care system. When wage controls imposed by the National War Labor Board prevented employers from competing for employees on the basis of wages, benefits became the main area of competition, and employers began offering comprehensive health insurance (Jacoby 1997, 216; Starr 1994, 60; Swenson and Greer 2002, 618). The tax system, which allowed employers to pay for health insurance without incurring payroll taxes, also encouraged employers to provide insurance and pay the premiums, as they were competing for scarce labor during the war. As the incentives of Obamacare continue to evolve, some scholars have argued that fewer employers will offer health insurance and will instead opt to encourage their employees to purchase affordable insurance on an individual basis (Emanuel 2014).

With the introduction of Medicare and Medicaid, the number of people receiving publicly funded health care rose dramatically. When the programs became law in 1965, Paul Starr noted that "some physicians initially swore they would organize a boycott, until cooler heads prevailed in the AMA [American Medical Association] and, after it went into effect a year later, the profession not only accepted Medicare but discovered it was a bonanza" (Starr 1982, 369–70), but Medicaid has remained detested by the medical profession.

Medicare and Medicaid provided access for health care for those over sixty-five years of age and for the poorest Americans, but the programs did not initially alter the system of health care provision for the majority of citizens. The seeds for the next transition were planted in the early 1970s, although that transition proved to be very gradual. Dr. Sidney Garfield, cofounder with Henry Kaiser of Kaiser Permanente, reflected on the stress on the health care system in the 1970s: "The US system of high-quality but expensive and poorly distributed medical care is in trouble. Dramatic advances in medical knowledge and new techniques, combined with soaring demands . . . are swamping the system by which medical care is delivered. As the disparity between the capabilities of medical care and its availability increases, and as costs rise beyond the ability of most Americans to pay them, pressures build up for action. High on the list of suggested remedies are national health insurance and a new medical care delivery system" (Debley 2009, 120). These thoughts addressing the problems of access, cost, and quality apply equally well to the crisis in health care that led to the Affordable Care Act of 2010. Ultimately the rise to dominance of managed care altered access to medical care for tens of millions of Americans. The key aspect of managed care, as opposed to conventional insurance, is its repositioning of decision-making power. Rather than patients or doctors determining who has access to which services, the discretion lies with the Health Maintenance Organization (HMO). Although this dramatically affected access to care, the affect on the delivery of care has been a little more complex.

With the failure of the Clinton-attempted health care reform of the 1990s, new vehicles emerged through which insurers hoped to deter "patients rights" bills that would increase the power of patients to require expenditures by their HMOs. In particular, the rise of the Preferred Provider Organization (PPO) gave the appearance of offering greater patient choice while actually offering employers flexibility to reduce choice and costs with plans "less subject to regulatory strictures" than HMOs (Hurley, Strunk, and White 2004, 56).

The HMOs have existed since the early twentieth century. They were initially founded as a way for workers and their bosses to prepay for health care, and they have traditionally had some advantages over other forms of health insurance coverage. In the best case scenario, HMOs may be well structured for providing integrated, continuous care. From the early 1970s, the federal government encouraged the use of HMOS, and the institutions experienced massive growth, both in the number of HMOs and in the number of HMO members (McNeil and Schlenker 1975). The HMOs received a massive boost in 1973 with the passage of the HMO Act. The act provided grants and loans to HMOs and required most employers to offer their employees an HMO plan if such a plan were available (Davis, Collins, and Morris 1994, 180).

About 20 percent of workers in the United States covered by employer-sponsored health care are in HMOs, although this number masks considerable regional variation. In the western United States, in 2009 about one-third of those with employment-based health insurance were in HMOs; in the Midwest the figure is far lower (Henry J. Kaiser Family Foundation 2009, 56). Medicare beneficiaries can also choose to receive their health care through HMOs. As of 2009, approximately 6.5 million Medicare beneficiaries (or around 45 million total beneficiaries) were receiving their benefits through an HMO (Henry J. Kaiser Family Foundation 2009). The most recent data from 2008 show that about 33.5 million Medicaid enrollees (approximately one-half of all enrollees) were receiving their benefits though an HMO (Centers for Medicare and Medicaid Services 2008).

Evolution of the UK System

The welfare institutions in the United Kingdom came into existence in their current form immediately after World War II. Although there were some welfare programs in place before 1945, they were not yet underpinned by the ideology of universal entitlement. The pre–World War II programs provided very little to very few; only the absolute neediest of citizens received any form of public assistance. The now classic report by William Beveridge (1942), commissioned by a Labour minister in the wartime national unity government, set out the principles of a universal welfare state offering "cradle to grave" care, and it quickly acquired the "status of a biblical text" (Glennerster 2000, 82). With the post–World War II welfare state came an understanding of welfare as a system of universal entitlements, through which the government would improve the standard of living for all of its citizens. Means testing was absent from almost all the new programs, and the well-off as well as the poor benefited from the new welfare institutions. Universal health care was at the center of the new welfare state.

The NHS was established by the National Health Service Act of 1946 and officially began operating in 1948 under the stewardship of Aneurin Bevan, the Minister of Health, who was a passionate proponent of universalized health care. In a pamphlet explaining the new health service to the general public at its launch, the NHS was described as follows: "It will provide you with all medical, dental, and nursing care. Everyone—rich or poor, man, woman or child—can use it or any part of it. There are no charges, except for a few special items. There are no insurance qualifications. But it is not a charity. You are all paying for it, mainly as taxpayers, and it will relieve your money worries in time of illness" (Central Office of Information for the Ministry of Health 1948, quoted in Webster 2002, 24).

The principle of NHS care being "free at the point of delivery" (i.e., paid for through general taxation) was part of the original rhetoric of the service, and it has become an article of faith in British politics (Jones 1994, 151). The NHS was very heavily used from the outset, even by those who could afford private health care, and the costs were much higher than anticipated (Glennerster 2000, 50, 79).

With the creation of the NHS came the consolidation of health-related employment with the government as employer. Those working in the health sector before the NHS had been employed under a variety of arrangements, ranging from volunteers and employees in charity hospitals to self-employed doctors, who worked on a private, fee-for-service basis. Under the new system, the state was the employer, and the pay rates were determined nationally.[1]

The British Medical Association (BMA) was a relatively strong organization that had been representing doctors long before the founding of the NHS. It was therefore the primary group representing the interests of the crucial employees (then potential employees) to the government during the process of creating the NHS. Scholarly accounts have often emphasized the role of doctors and their professional associations in creating and constraining national health care institutions (Immergut 1992). The BMA was founded in 1832 and had been active for over a century before the issue of a comprehensive national health service was realistically under discussion. In 1930 (and again in 1938) the BMA had drawn up its own proposal for a "general medical service." In principle, then, the BMA was not against the idea of universal or near-universal health care provision. This stance contrasts with the American Medical Association's position on universal coverage, which it has not advocated since 1913. The BMA, however, strongly opposed (and very nearly defeated) the NHS as set forth in the 1946 act, out of concern for the "effects on the livelihood of practitioners" (British Medical Association 1997). Indeed, "the BMA led outright opposition to the scheme and opposed the official plan both in principle and in detail" (Glennerster 2000, 44).

Although at first refusing to sign on to the government's proposal, the BMA ultimately acquiesced after receiving concessions regarding the terms and conditions of doctors' employment. Most significantly, the doctors were

---

1. The exception is general practitioners (GPs or family doctors), who are legally self-employed and contracted to the National Health Service.

allowed to continue to treat private patients, thus supplementing their NHS income. This concession was referred to by Bevan as "stuffing their mouths with gold" as the change in policy essentially bought the acquiescence of the BMA (Irvine 2001). Although Bevan claimed he would proceed with the introduction of the NHS regardless of the cooperation of the BMA, it is difficult to imagine that this could have ever worked in practice. From the very beginning of the NHS, then, employee interests have been central. Once the NHS was established, it was not its existence that was questioned by employees but the mechanisms for the delivery of health care and the terms and conditions of employment for its staff. One history of the first fifty years of the NHS aptly described its state as one of "continuous revolution" (Webster 2002, 140).

Stakeholders

The US Scenario

As in the United Kingdom and in all health care systems, the key stakeholders in the US health care economy are payers, patients, providers, and government. The roles of and relationships among these stakeholders are more complex in the United States than in the United Kingdom because of the fragmented, mixed economy of US health care and the role of insurance companies as intermediaries.

The patients, as in all countries, are those who use health care, and in the United States their interests are often mediated through, and distorted by, health insurers. The other groups of stakeholders are much more fragmented. The health care payers are the individuals and organizations that pay for health care. This payment may be mediated by insurers or HMOs (which were originally known as prepaid health plans), or it may be direct. The cost of health care is covered in the United States either by the individual, an employer, or the government. Some individuals buy their own health insurance or pay per service when they need health care. Before the implementation of the ACA, about 8 percent of the nonelderly population of the United States, about 14 million people, purchased their own private health insurance, primarily because they were ineligible for any government- or employer-sponsored coverage (Henry J. Kaiser Family Foundation 2010, 1).

Although the data are still somewhat unclear, the best estimates are that around 4 million people now have purchased new individual or family (not employer-sponsored) health insurance primarily via the ACA health insurance exchanges (Sanger-Katz 2014).

The majority of the nonelderly US population receives their health insurance from an employer or the employer of a family member. Around 71 percent of the population is covered by employer-sponsored health insurance, a number that has remained steady since the implementation of the ACA (Blavin et al. 2015). The rest of the population is either uninsured (about 17 percent of the population) or covered by a government health care or health insurance program. The main government programs are the reimbursement/insurance programs: Medicare for those over 65 years of age and Medicaid for low-income Americans.

Although the largest proportion of health care in the United States is delivered by the private sector, there are some public sector health care providers. It is difficult to calculate the proportion of all health care employment that is in the public sector; however, including both frontline health care workers and administrators, probably about 5 percent of health care employment is in the public sector (University of Michigan Center of Excellence in Public Health Workforce Studies 2013). The public employers include public hospitals, prison health care clinics and hospitals, hospitals owned and operated by the Indian Health Service and the Veterans Health Administration, and Department of Defense health care facilities for active members of the military. There is direct federal provision of health care for certain eligible veterans through the Veterans Health Administration and for American Indians and Alaska Natives though the Indian Health Service. The Veterans Health Administration and the Indian Health Service are programs operated by the government as both payer and provider, whereas Medicaid and Medicare are systems for public payment but private provision of health care.

These payers all have a vested interest in keeping costs down, but otherwise their interests are quite diffuse. For example, an employer may wish to ensure that its workforce is healthy, but it is unlikely to be invested in ensuring long-term health. On the other hand, an injured veteran who receives health care from the Veterans Administration (VA) is likely to use the VA as his primary health care provider for the rest of his life. The VA thus has an interest in covering preventive care and in taking a long-term view of a patient's well-being. The health services are all publicly owned and operated agencies that deliver health care to prescribed groups of citizens. They differ from the voucher programs (Medicare and Medicaid) in that they are actual health care systems rather than reimbursement mechanisms. Medicare and Medicaid are government health insurance programs rather than government health care delivery programs. The model of publicly funded and publicly provided health care is most directly comparable to the UK NHS but makes up a small fraction of the whole US health care economy.

In addition to the single-payer, single-provider health care agencies in the United States, there are also publicly owned clinics and hospitals, community health centers, and various public health programs. These organizations provide health care to a diverse set of patients: the uninsured, those on public programs such as Medicaid, and often some who are insured. Publicly owned and operated hospitals tend to operate as safety net hospitals, providing care to those who cannot get health care anywhere else. The ACA also significantly incentivized the formation of Accountable Care Organizations (ACOs), which integrate hospitals and doctors into single organizations and, theoretically, share the savings that should result from higher quality preventative care (Gold 2014). The ACOs and medical homes, similar to the longstanding structure of Kaiser Permanente, seek to emphasize investment in primary care such as diabetes prevention in order to save money on acute care (Silberner 2011).

The UK Scenario

The key stakeholders in the NHS have remained relatively stable since its founding. The payers, providers, and patients all operate within a unitary, national structure. For the patient, the system is essentially seamless. Each patient registers with a local primary care doctor and can receive specialist treatment from a local hospital or elsewhere in the country if more specialized care is required. All health care provision and health care employment are overseen by the Department of Health, run by both politicians and nonpolitical civil servants. In theory (although not always in practice), the employment practices as well as the clinical practices should be the same anywhere in the country.

Financial Structures

The US Payment System

The influence of the CMS in structuring health care delivery should not be underestimated. As DeWalt et al. emphasized, "CMS finances health care for more Americans than any other single entity." The number of health care recipients whose care is indirectly regulated by the CMS dwarfs the number of Medicare and Medicaid recipients, and many hospitals treat all patients according to CMS rules; in other words, "clinical medicine has become intertwined with CMS" (DeWalt et al. 2005–6, 79). In the current health care economy, "most private and public insurers base their payments on Medicare fee schedules and regulations" (Hariri et al. 2007). Medicare is not simply a health insurance program for older Americans; it is the structuring principle behind all health care delivery and payment in the United States: "Medicare has a considerable impact on the American health-care system not just because it comprises a substantial portion of health-care provider payments but also because of the ripple effects of the program's policies on other health-care delivery systems. The Medicare fee schedule has become the de facto national health-care reimbursement schedule for all physician services" (Hariri et al. 2007).

In the 2009–10 debate over health care reform, problems with payment structures and perverse incentives in the fee-for-service system were consistently at the forefront of the discussion. An article in the *New Yorker* by Atul Gawande, a physician, made a forceful case for reforming health care through realigning the incentives for physicians (Gawande 2009b). The article focused on McAllen, Texas, a town with extraordinarily high health care costs, as determined by the Dartmouth Health Atlas (Dartmouth Institute for Health Policy and Clinical Practice 2010). Gawande emphatically demonstrated that when physicians' income depends not only on the quantity of service provided but on ownership of equipment and facilities, the relationship between cost and quality goes into free fall. Gawande's article heavily influenced President Obama's reform proposals and "became required reading in the White House" (Pear 2009). Ultimately this concern did not translate into a shift in health care financing or the incentives for physicians but in separate nods to comparative effectiveness research and cost containment in the 2010 act (Patient-Centered Outcomes Research Institute 2014).

The key purchasers of health care in the United States are health insurance companies. Most individuals have health insurance, usually subsidized by an employer, through which they procure all or most of their health care. Insurers, therefore, wield a great deal of power. Insurers determine who can receive what care and who can provide what care. Health insurance companies are essentially health care brokers.

Starr (1982, 291) categorizes health insurance plans as offering indemnity benefits, partial reimbursement for health care expenses, service benefits with direct payment to the health care provider, or direct services that provide health care directly from the insurance company to the individual provider or member. The latter category includes the HMO model, such as Kaiser Permanente, where members are essentially buying into a closed system of health care payment and service provision. Starr points out that these types of plan give the insurer a very different role in mediating between the patient and the health care provider. Direct service plans give the insurer the most discretion in the form and quantity of care available to an individual. In response to rising health care costs in the 1920s, these health insurance plans burgeoned in the 1930s.

Blue Cross plans were founded and controlled by hospitals, essentially controlling prices and providing group discounts for members (Enthoven 1993; Starr 1982). When the plans moved from single hospitals to large city or regionwide groupings, they "effectively became monopolies in hospital prepayment" (Starr 1982, 297), discouraging rather than encouraging competition on the basis of cost. Blue Shield plans were analogous to the Blue Cross plans but were controlled by physicians rather than hospitals (Enthoven 1993; Starr 1982). Both of the so-called Blues required enabling legislation at the state level, and in many states these plans dominated the state insurance landscape for decades.

In the 1930s and 1940s the Blue plans dominated nationally, but by the 1950s commercial, indemnity-style plans began to surpass them in raw subscriber numbers. In the late 1940s and 1950s, the number of Americans with employer-sponsored health insurance plans increased rapidly, as did the number purchasing individual insurance. This trend continued into the 1970s when HMOs took center stage. By the 1980s, the now merged Blue Cross Blue Shield Association could no longer make the case that it was a not-for-profit organization. The leaders of the association acknowledged that, since the early days when their nonprofit status was initially determined, the plans had evolved into more businesslike corporations. Ultimately a special tax status was created for the Blue Cross Blue Shield Association, treating it neither fully as a nonprofit nor a for-profit organization and applying significant new taxes to the association (Cunningham and Cunningham 1997).[2]

Public Health Services in the United Kingdom

In the United Kingdom, the NHS is funded from general taxation, including payroll taxes. From its earliest days, Bevan and other NHS proponents insisted on a service that was "free at the point of use." The founders were careful to present the system as not "free" or costless, but rather as a system without direct usage charges. As demand soared after 1948, the service introduced some charges for prescriptions for employed patients and for some dental and eye care services. These are somewhat analogous to the small co-pays common in US health insurance plans. In the 1980s, the hospitals were restructured as "trusts," entities consisting of a small number of existing hospital sites (or primary care groups) with some degree of managerial autonomy. Under the Blair government in the 2000s, some hospital trusts were granted even more autonomy through "foundation" status to reward their high performance ratings. Although now more services, especially support services, are provided to the NHS by private companies (see chapter 5), the single payer remains the government.

The Workplaces

In the United States

The American hospital workplace features an unusual set of employment relationships. The professional hierarchy mimics that of hospitals across the

---

2. Blue Cross and Blue Shield were initially structurally different from other insurance companies because they set their costs through "community rating" and were structured as nonprofit rather than for-profit companies. However, the competition from companies using conventional experience rating rather than community rating ultimately made the Blues drop their unusual, less costly approach (Robinson 2003).

industrialized world, but the group at the top of the hierarchy is composed of freelancers, not employees. The tradition of physicians working physically in hospitals but outside the organization creates an exaggerated version of the usual hierarchy in health care.

The hospital workplace is regulated by the complex patchwork of voluntary and mandatory agencies mentioned earlier. The workplace challenges consistently mentioned by health care workers are present in hospitals in both the United States and the United Kingdom, but employees and their representatives face a choice of whether to try to address problems in the workplace through collective bargaining or other employer-level mechanisms or through legislation on either the state or federal level.

In raw employment numbers, health care is both the largest and the fastest growing industry in the United States. Over 18 million people work in the health care industry in the U.S. (US Bureau of Labor Statistics 2015).[3] Of these, around 3 million are RNs (U.S. Department of Health and Human Services, Health Resources and Services Administration, and National Center for Health Workforce Analysis 2014; US Health Resources and Services Administration 2010). Hospitals employ about one-third of U.S. health care workers (this figure excludes doctors, who usually are not employees of hospitals even when they practice primarily in hospitals). Just under a third of hospital employees are RNs, with additional hospital staff working in nursing-related occupations in roles defined as, for example, licensed practical nurses, licensed vocational nurses, nursing aides, or certified nursing assistants (US Bureau of Labor Statistics 2010).[4]

There are currently about 650,000 physicians working in the United States, and the number is projected to rise by about 20 percent by 2018 (US Bureau of Labor Statistics 2009). As of 2008, primary care physicians had a median income of about $220,000; the figure for specialists was about $396,000 (US Bureau of Labor Statistics 2014). Physician compensation is the

---

3. There are no perfect data for measuring the size of the US health care workforce. Measuring workers by industry may miss many people who work in health care; for example, public sector health care workers may be classified as working in public administration, and those who work in health insurance administration are likely to be classified as working in the insurance rather than the health care industry. Although it is impossible to exactly quantify the number of people working directly or indirectly in health care, it is likely that the figure is significantly higher than 14 million.

4. Due to cuts to the US Bureau of Labor Statistics, more recent data are not available.

subject of much debate and controversy, and this pay differential is frequently blamed for the current shortage of primary care doctors (Steinbrook 2009). It is important to note that there are a number of unusual aspects to the employment relationship for specialist physicians. Many specialist physicians are self-employed and maintain practicing privileges at one or more hospitals. Physicians must maintain a high level of malpractice insurance and often bear some of the costs of operating an office or other practice facilities and equipment. Many doctors also accrue a great deal of debt for their medical education, which they must then repay.

The evolution of the medical profession in the United States has been superbly recounted elsewhere, most notably by Starr (1982). For the purposes of this account, it is necessary to touch only briefly upon both the development of the profession and of the major organizations representing physicians in the workplace and beyond. Some scholars have examined the role of physicians and their associations in shaping health care systems in the United States and beyond, but these authors tend to minimize the significance of doctors in the health care workplace (Immergut 1992). It is impossible to understand the evolution or contemporary configuration of the US health care economy without understanding the role of doctors. "In the twentieth century, not only did physicians become a powerful, prestigious, and wealthy profession, but they succeeded in shaping the basic organization and financial structure of American medicine" (Starr 1982, 8).

Starr addresses, in great detail, the origins and consolidation of professional sovereignty and autonomy in medicine. As in most advanced industrialized countries, the medical profession is heavily regulated (or self-regulated), and professional judgment and discretion are central to the practice of the profession. Starr has argued, "The profession has been able to turn its authority into social privilege, economic power and political influence. In the distribution of rewards from medicine, the medical profession, as the highest-paid occupation in our society, receives a radically disproportionate share" (Starr 1982, 5). Presently, only about a quarter of physicians receive a fixed salary; the vast majority are either compensated on a fee-for-service basis with performance incentives, through ownership of their practices, or by some combination of all three (Boukus, Cassil, and O'Malley 2009).

The vast majority of doctors practicing in a hospital are labeled "voluntary." They are not hospital employees but have admitting and practicing privileges within the hospital (there are often a small number of hospitalists—directly employed physicians who administer care for in-patients). This unusual employment arrangement complicates the workplace dynamic in hospitals, where in addition to the status hierarchy (often engendering status anxiety), doctors have autonomy and are operating outside the conventional employment relationship. While nursing staff provide continuity of care, physicians have much more fleeting involvement in patient care.

Although nursing became an institutionalized profession later than medicine, it followed the classic path toward professionalization. Sioban Nelson (2001) has documented the early history of nursing as a profession in the nineteenth century. This argument demonstrates the strong similarities in the early development of nursing in multiple national contexts. In the nineteenth century, the advanced industrial countries had similar health care systems consisting of some private fee-for-service provision and much charitable provision of care. Nelson also points to the lasting influence of the British empire in shaping the role of nurses in former British colonies. Over time, the nursing profession has become more institutionalized and is subject to licensing and credentialing requirements (which vary by state). With licensing and therefore entry to the profession controlled by the states, it is no surprise that state nursing associations were key to the early union representation of American nurses.

About 19.8 percent of RNs are members of unions (Clark 2013). More than a dozen unions represent nurses, from the nurse-only unions such as the California Nurses Association/National Nurses United, to an array of unions traditionally associated with different industries, such as the American Federation of Teachers, the United Auto Workers, and the United Steelworkers. Some unions strongly believe in nurse-only unions and nurse-only bargaining units while others, most notably the Service Employees International Union, strive to represent all health care workers in a given workplace. As I discuss more extensively in chapter 6, nurse unions operate at both the workplace and the legislative level. The depth and quality of workplace representation varies considerably.

The American Nurses Association (ANA), a professional association founded in 1911, has been closely linked with the credentialing of nurses in the United States. The ANA has always claimed to represent all the nurses in the United States, but in reality there has been a great deal of internal strife within the organization. In 1999, some state-level ANA affiliates formed United American Nurses (UAN), a union focused on nurse organizing and collective bargaining (Gordon 2009, 281). Many state nurses associations became dissatisfied with their representation through UAN/ANA and particularly with their lack of control over their dues. Most notably, the California Nurses Association (CNA) split from UAN/ANA in 1995 and began to organize nurses much more aggressively. The CNA won a lengthy campaign to mandate minimum nurse–patient ratios throughout California, and this law has served as a model for campaigns in other states (Gordon, Buchanan, and Bretherton 2008). The CNA, and its national union, National Nurses United, has consistently argued that the ANA represents management nurses and administrators, while the CNA and its allies represent bedside nurses.

The complex landscape of nurse unionism in the United States reflects the complex landscape of health care employment. In some cases, unions that were regionally powerful reached out to local nurses. In others, unions saw nursing as a growth area and seized the opportunity to organize well-paid workers in a healthy sector of the economy. In some cases, unions represent all or most employees under a given employer; for instance, the American Federation of Government Employees represents nurses within the VA (as well as other professional and nonprofessional VA workers). To present a strong legislative front, the American Federation of Labor-Congress of Industrial Organizations (AFL-CIO) created an umbrella group, RNs Working Together, comprising the ten AFL-CIO–affiliated unions that represent nurses (AFL-CIO 2007). This loose group, however, did very little as a coordinated coalition because a few major unions dominate nursing representation and the competition over new nurse organizing is fierce.

In the United Kingdom

Employing more than 1.6 million people in 2010, the NHS is one of the largest employers in the world and the largest employer in the United Kingdom. The biggest occupational group in the service is nurses, who make up about just under a third of the workforce. There are about 125,000 doctors in the NHS (including both family doctors and hospital-based specialists). The majority of these staff are members of unions, many of which also function as professional associations, and their pay and conditions are determined either by collective bargaining or collective consultation. The largest unions in the NHS are the Royal College of Nursing, the British Medical Association, and UNISON, but there are around twenty unions representing NHS staff. All public employees in Britain are eligible for union membership and collective bargaining coverage, and many senior managers are represented by UNISON. Union density in health care hovers around 50 percent, with coverage (in the form of collective pay determination) considerably higher (Bach, Givan, and Forth 2009, 318).

The Department of Health has embraced a partnership-based approach to the creation of NHS policy, particularly as it affects health service staff. Because staff deliver the services, any changes to NHS policy necessitate the cooperation of frontline staff and managers. This strategy acknowledges the potential difficulties in implementing policy without the acquiescence of employees.

Civil servants at the highest level of government recognize the role of good management practice in improving overall health service quality. The Department of Health is primarily staffed by civil servants, with politicians holding the positions of secretary of state (the top, cabinet-level position) and ministers (the more junior positions). Some of the civil servants are career bureaucrats, but the most senior staff tend to have experience in health care administration or delivery; for example, the chief medical officer is a doctor, the chief nursing officer is a credentialed nurse, and the director and deputy directors of human resources usually have experience in NHS management at the local level. These civil servants are responsible for advising ministers and the secretary of state on issues of both legislation and regulation. These ministers and civil servants are responsible for both regulating and administering the NHS—the largest unitary health system in the world.

Although changes in health policy tend to be politically driven, civil servants are able to advise on issues such as public health and efficiency. While elected politicians may choose key policy objectives, civil servants select the best way to meet these objectives. Because all NHS services are delivered by staff, the Human Resources Directorate at the Department of Health plays a crucial role in the reform process. In this sense, staffing issues permeate every aspect of institutional reform in the NHS. The directorate is responsible for human resources across the NHS and must ensure that there is effective and appropriate staffing throughout the organization. Proactive human resource initiatives from the Department of Health have included a policy to coordinate the ethical recruitment of nurses and doctors from abroad (so as not to poach from developing countries suffering from their own staffing crises) and new procedures for staff training and development (personal interviews 2002–5).

The Department of Health civil servants interviewed for this book all took their roles as advocates of the public interest very seriously. Although most expressed confidence that the objectives of the current government and the methods for meeting these objectives were the most appropriate ones, all were aware of the potential for tension between immediate political objectives and longer-term public health goals. These civil servants saw themselves as objective and as being above the special interests and infighting of health service managers and employee groups.

The civil servants did express the concern that health service providers and their unions and professional associations were sometimes overly self-interested and protectionist, and therefore reluctant to change. One spoke about the obstacles in the way of pay and job restructuring because of rigid professional boundaries and historical job classifications. The civil servants justified the imposition of unpopular policies by focusing on long-term strategic health care objectives. These civil servants were also convinced that people are central to the functioning of the NHS, and they used the rhetoric of partnership and incremental, evidence-based change to discuss creative ways to move beyond the obstacles. Overcoming employee rigidities is a key element of the work of the human resources directorate (various personal interviews, 2002).

The media can sometimes put pressure on the government when a particular negative incident has occurred. Three of the four Members of Parliament (MPs) interviewed stated that they would not encourage their constituents to go to the media until all other avenues for resolving the particular problem had been fully explored. These MPs were sympathetic to the difficult work of NHS staff and felt that media pressure and criticism were not helpful in improving the performance of the NHS, although one did acknowledge that media pressure could sometimes be helpful in obtaining the desired response or reaction from either the national government or the local health service provider involved. One Conservative MP was the only interviewee who felt that NHS staff were sometime overly concerned with their own interests rather than the interests of the NHS as a whole. All others expressed sympathy for the difficult work and low pay of NHS staff. The Conservative Party, traditionally at odds with public sector unions, stated on its web site that "we will set the NHS free from ministerial meddling and allow NHS staff to concentrate on doing what they do best: providing top-quality care to patients" (Conservative Party 2009).

I interviewed MPs about NHS restructuring and asked whether they heard particular concerns from the NHS staff among their constituents (personal interviews 2002). The two MPs from relatively high cost-of-living areas said they heard frequently that NHS pay (particularly for nurses) was inadequate. One stated that "I do get letters from people who are nurses telling me why they don't want to be nurses any longer, and they say things like they can get more money stacking cans in [a supermarket]." Another stated that he heard frequent complaints from NHS employees: "not enough equipment, unhappy with the pay that they're receiving, feeling that the distortion of waiting list priorities means that they're not doing their job as well as perhaps they would like. Complaining about training, you name it." The MPs were acutely aware of the concerns for staff that are key causes of recruitment and retention problems. At the same time, all felt that other areas of the NHS were also underfunded, and that increased funding of the NHS should not primarily raise wages.

Health issues in general and the NHS specifically remain "intensely political" in the United Kingdom (Berridge 1999, 98). In this section I briefly highlight four key forms of restructuring that pervade both policymaking and implementation in the process of NHS reform: the shortage of skilled staff; workforce restructuring (and, to some extent, flexibilization); the process of decentralization and devolution of authority; and the financing of public services, including private sector involvement.

As the NHS is one of the world's largest employers, any management initiative in the organization must trickle down to a large number of frontline staff before any change is realized. In recent years, the role of human resource management in this process has been taken much more seriously throughout the organization. Politicians and health care leaders have begun to speak of "change fatigue," in reference to the constant attempts to implement change in the health service. In a sense, then, continuity in the NHS means continuous change. It is almost impossible to pinpoint the start and end of the ongoing waves of reform. The main restructuring initiatives since the late 1990s fall into four main categories, with some overlap between the categories. The first area, human resource management, follows the trend across the public and private sectors with an emphasis on routinizing best practices for people management. Examples of these practices include staff development and appraisal, a focus on employee voice and staff involvement, and initiatives to improve flexibility and work-life balance for employees. The second area of major restructuring is in pay—both in the system of individual pay determination (within a collectively bargained structure) and in overall pay levels determined nationally. Examples of pay restructuring include a new collectively bargained contract for doctors and the job evaluation framework for other NHS staff, known as Agenda for Change. The third major area of change is the rise of performance monitoring. Since the 1990s, NHS hospital managers have been required to report on a wide range of performance outcomes and the degree to which their hospital has implemented government-mandated procedures. All NHS trusts must also survey their patients and staff regularly. These metrics are used to rate the hospitals. The final category of restructuring is the rise of subcontracting and privatization of services. This includes subcontracting so-called hotel services such as cleaning and catering, but also contracting with private companies to provide entire clinics that perform elective and diagnostic procedures to NHS patients.

The emphasis on improved human resources practices as a route to improving all aspects of health care has been embraced from the very highest level of government. As one senior civil servant with responsibility for NHS human resources put it, "My fundamental belief is that if you look after staff better and help staff to get the best out of themselves, that's likely to benefit patients too" (personal interview 2002). This commitment to best practice human resources and the centrality of human resources in performance targets was something of a relief to workplace human resources directors because they no longer had to explain to their chief executives why these functions were so crucial. The core of the emerging human resources initiatives was first summarized in *HR in the NHS plan*, a report issued in 2002 (National Workforce Taskforce, and HR Directorate 2002). The report highlighted four areas in which improved human resources practices and new initiatives could improve the performance of NHS hospitals. The key areas were making the NHS a model employer, providing clear career paths through a so-called skills escalator, improving staff morale, and building management skills (National Workforce Taskforce, and HR Directorate

2002, 7). These strategies all conform to the goal of improving the experience and quality of the workforce while also improving efficiency and clinical outcomes.

Under the banner of "more staff, working differently," the Department of Health began paying particular attention to management practices, which might improve both patient care and the workplace experience of staff. A few of the reform initiatives were brought about in response to European Union–level directives (particularly the reduction in hours for junior doctors), but most were simply an attempt to improve overall outcomes. There were a number of enforcement mechanisms for the local implementation of these practices, primarily related to the audit and monitoring procedures. There were numerous initiatives that local mangers were required to implement, and only a sampling are discussed here.

One of the earliest of the New Labor–era human resources initiatives, Improving Working Lives, was essentially a checklist launched in 2001 that laid out specific areas in which hospitals could improve the lives of their employees through initiatives such as more flexible working hours and greater staff involvement in decision making. Hospitals were initially encouraged to achieve the standard of Improving Working Lives with a three-year deadline for mandatory compliance. The standards covered a range of areas from diversity policies to work–life balance. Although the best run organizations were likely to be achieving these standards without the initial pressure of monitoring, the guidance to less well-managed hospitals was clear and specific. The standards conformed to traditional human resource management models, encouraging the up-skilling of staff, ongoing training and appraisal, and flexible work opportunities. A key objective of Improving Working Lives was to create a better, happier, healthier workforce and to realize these benefits in improved care and more satisfied patients. The human resources literature supported the contention that these policies would improve retention of staff (Givan, Avgar, and Liu 2010).

There was also an effort to reassess the appropriate skills for key tasks in health care provision and, where possible, to assign tasks to less skilled (and easier to recruit) employees. A prime example of this is the role of the health care assistant (Bach, Kessler, and Heron 2008). Health care assistants now perform many of the tasks previously reserved for RNs, including personal hygiene, moving and handling, and phlebotomy. The NHS has also undertaken a massive job evaluation exercise under the heading of Agenda for Change in order to increase flexibility (beyond professional boundaries) and ensure that staff are paid appropriately (Department of Health 2003a). The quest for increased staff development and training, however, is ongoing, and dramatic changes have yet to be fully realized (Buchan and Evans 2007).

The response to staff shortage also dovetails with the key goal of those in the Department of Health's Human Resources Directorate: "More staff, working differently" (National Workforce Taskforce, and HR Directorate 2002). The working differently aspect is addressed by the Agenda for Change initiative and also by the concept of the skills escalator, which was central to the mission of Andrew Foster, who served as Director of Human Resources at the Department of Health (see, for example, Foster 2002). Foster argued that skill flexibility and up-skilling of those with low skills in the NHS would improve the quality of service.

The devolution of management power to the workplace could theoretically mean more freedom over terms and conditions of employment, although this has so far been a sticking point for the unions. Although foundation hospitals were thought more likely to "offer new rewards and explore innovative ways of working" (Department of Health 2002b, 40), concerns about the poaching of staff for the professions with shortages and about the nationally agreed pay restructuring under Agenda for Change also applying to foundation trusts have limited the actual effect of these so-called freedoms on employment conditions. The strategy of decentralization has been heavily constrained by the interests of employees (including managers).

The 2012 Health and Social Care Act relocated financial and decision-making powers in the NHS. The "biggest revolution in the NHS for 60 years" created Clinical Commissioning Groups of primary care practices, which have responsibility for purchasing all care for their patients. This massive program of change was not announced by the Conservative party during the 2010 election campaign, and it was opposed by all the major professional associations and unions representing doctors (*BMJ* Editors 2011). Clare Gerada, the chair of the Royal College of General Practitioners, which was the organized interest group of professionals ostensibly being granted key decision-making powers by this reform, cautioned that, with these changes, "the government's proposals run a risk of destabilizing the NHS and causing long-term harm to patient outcomes" (*BMJ* Editors 2011). In this case of top-down reform, even those frontline workers being granted significant power to determine the shape of health care delivery disavowed both the process and direction of change.

Although these policy innovations could dramatically reshape the NHS, the actions of employees and their representative organizations make radical change unlikely. The staff and unions make the institutions of the NHS extremely "sticky" and slow to change. As the history of the NHS shows, its employees, who are essential to its functioning, are generally conservative and reluctant to change in any but the most incremental ways, and the response of NHS staff to major policy initiatives is the critical determinant of their successful implementation.

Chapter 2

Turbulence in the Two Systems

The Political Impulse for Change in the United States

Between the 1970s and the 1990s, managed care came to dominate the American health care landscape. Medicare and Medicaid covered the older and poor populations, respectively, and most Americans received health insurance through their employer or the employer of a family member. The number of uninsured people, however, rose steadily from the 1970s to the 1990s (Gilmer and Kronick 2001; Kronick and Gilmer 1999). Rising health care costs and the increasing number of uninsured people were a major issue in the 1992 presidential election, when Bill Clinton, running against the incumbent President George H. W. Bush, vowed to bring sweeping health care reform to the country, if elected.

Bill Clinton's 1992 presidential campaign initially focused on vaguely formulated ideas about health care reform, such as guaranteeing health care security for all (Hacker 1997; Skocpol 1995). Paul Starr, the sociologist who became part of Clinton's health care reform team, argued that "uncontrolled growth in costs and deepening insecurities about insurance are not only problems in health care; they are also an index of political failure" (Starr 1994, 27). Working with a team of political advisors and policy experts, Clinton gradually refined the reform proposal to emphasize "regional insurance purchasing agencies along with modest new tax subsidies to push the employer-based U.S. health care system toward cost efficiency and universal coverage" (Skocpol 1995, 69).

Clinton's plan of increasing regulation to foster "managed competition" was a kind of middle ground, ostensibly designed to rein in costs without creating undue government interference either in health care markets or employee benefits decisions. Once in office, President Clinton appointed his wife, Hillary Rodham Clinton, to lead the White House's effort to reform health care as the head of a twelve-person task force. Because this followed closely on the heels of the three-way presidential election focused on the problems caused by the budget deficit, balancing the budget was a key priority. It seemed politically impossible to propose a health care reform package that would increase deficit spending, so the Clinton plan focused on increased coverage paired with cost control. These themes re-emerged in President Barack Obama's plan for health care reform during and after the 2008 presidential election.

Hacker (1997, 171) argued that "Clinton and his advisers embraced managed competition within a budget precisely because they believed that it stood a better chance than other comprehensive reform proposals of surviving the American political gauntlet." Another factor diminishing the chances of the proposal's success, according to Gottschalk, was division within organized labor, especially the ongoing debate over whether single-payer or an employer mandate was the solution, and this gave labor an inability to provide practical policy support to Clinton (Gottschalk 2000, 137–58).

The great irony of the failed Clinton reform is that it gave birth to a boom in managed care, without the attendant employer mandate that might have increased access and slowed the rise of the uninsured. Both before and after the Clinton reform effort, the political wrangling successfully illuminated many key problems with the health care and health insurance systems, but it failed to solve these problems. This spawned an industry of consultants and credentials, profiting from the sale of performance-improvement strategies to health care providers. These initiatives ranged from Magnet Hospital Status (first awarded by the American Nurses Credentialing Center in 1994) to the multibillion-dollar health care management consulting industry, which is growing at a rate of almost 20 percent a year (American Nurses Credentialing Center 2014; Sager 2013). From 1993 to 1996, the number of Americans whose health insurance was delivered through health maintenance organizations (HMOs) jumped from 21 to 31 percent of those with employer-sponsored insurance (Henry J. Kaiser Family Foundation 2005). The number of Americans now enrolled in HMO-based health care through Medicare, Medicaid, or employment-based insurance is around 75 million people and rising, according to the latest available data (Henry J. Kaiser Family Foundation 2015c).

Some of the oldest HMOs, such as Kaiser Permanente and Group Health of Puget Sound, are nonprofit organizations, but others are not. Some scholars have debated whether one form of ownership or another is more beneficial to either high-quality care or cost control. Some argue that the profit motive promotes competition and cost control; others argue that not-for-profits can focus on high-quality care without excessive emphasis on cost cutting. Robert Kuttner argued in 1998 that "one of the original promises of prepaid group health was to improve coordination of services. It is ironic, then, that despite a lot of talk about 'virtual staff models,' many nominal HMOs today are actually far-flung assortments of doctors with strict utilization controls or financial incentives but little ongoing interaction, much less a common approach to practice. For-profit plans are leading this trend, but some nonprofit plans are following suit because of competitive pressures" (Kuttner 1998, 1562). Although Kuttner made the observation over a decade ago, it is even more applicable today.

By the end of the Clinton presidency, it was clear that the health care crisis was only growing worse. Blumenthal (1999, 1916) observed that "we seem to be wrestling with many of the same health policy demons that occupied us in 1994 and, indeed, for thirty years before that: the large and growing number of uninsured Americans, the high overall costs of our health care system, and pervasive evidence of the suboptimal quality of care." The ongoing failure of the system to provide low-cost, high-quality health care available to all continued through the 2008 election. Indeed, costs were still rising, quality was still questionable (debates over which measures most effectively capture health care quality not withstanding), and the number of uninsured and underinsured Americans was rapidly rising.

As the health care crisis progressed from chronic to acute, health care was a dominant campaign issue in the 2008 presidential election. All the major candidates offered a proposal for health care reform. The key differences in the proposals addressed the degree of government involvement in health care insurance and the use of mandates—mandating employers to provide insurance, or mandating individuals to purchase insurance, or both. Other key proposals ran the gamut of the health care economy, from reforming tort laws in an attempt to lower the cost of malpractice insurance to regulating insurers to prohibit some of their most egregious actions. No major candidate proposed national health insurance or a single-payer or socialized system of any kind.

After taking office, Obama modified his proposals for health care reform. Opposition to change reached a fever pitch, culminating in the notorious Tea Party protests against government intervention at town meetings around the country in the summer of 2009 (Herszenhorn and Stolberg 2009; Urbina 2009). When it became clear that the Democrats could not pass a reform plan without compromise on the so-called public option, a service that would be similar to Medicare, Obama began to negotiate with the Republicans. Although Obama's plan incorporated a number of compromises along the way, it ultimately passed through Congress without any Republican support.

In the United States, one can see the push and pull between privatization and resistance in the rejection of a single-payer option in the Obamacare deliberation process. This apparent rejection of public funding actually led to the vast majority of newly insured Americans being covered by Medicaid, a massive public program. Change from below that pushes back against neoliberalism illustrates a dynamic that repeats again and again in both the United States and the United Kingdom. In the case of Obamacare, the pendulum swung in the direction of private provision and market-based health care.

The Patient Protection and Affordability Act of 2010 was the result of Obama's push for health care reform, passed only after protracted deal making and parliamentary maneuvers. The act was phased in gradually, with several key provisions delayed from the timelines set out in the original act. The act imposes requirements on individuals, employers, and insurance companies. Individuals must purchase insurance or pay a fine; if insurance is not available through an employer or through expanded Medicaid eligibility, they may purchase insurance through an "exchange" where private insurers offer plans. Lower income Americans who cannot afford insurance but do not meet Medicaid eligibility requirements have access to government subsidies for the purchase of private insurance. Employers with more than fifty employees are required to offer insurance to their employees or pay an additional payroll tax. The smallest employers receive a subsidy toward the cost of health insurance. Insurers are faced with a large set of new regulations, including the inability to deny coverage based on preexisting conditions, the prohibition of lifetime limits on insurance benefits, and a mandate to provide coverage in several areas, such as preventive care and mental health (Democratic Policy Committee 2010).

The crucial element in these reforms is that they increase access to care but do not necessarily change the delivery of care once the system is accessed by a patient. In other words, they do not affect the central argument here, which is about the change initiatives that affect the way in which health care is delivered. The key challenge to frontline health care providers will be to increase the capacity of the system and to contain costs (a much vaguer goal of the act). The actual mechanism for increasing capacity and containing costs is not fully specified (with the partial exception of the incentives provided for accountable care organizations and medical homes), so the power of consultants and changes pushed from above remains untrammeled (Sager 2013).

Restructuring in the United Kingdom

The basic structures of the NHS remained generally unchanged from the service's founding until the Thatcher governments of the 1980s. From the Thatcher era to the present, the major exception to this has been in the area of pay, which has been the subject of repeated attempts at restructuring (and attacks on collective bargaining). The NHS had always been highly centralized, but Thatcher's Conservative government strongly advocated decentralization across the public services. The major change under Thatcher was the creation of self-governing NHS trusts with some autonomy over organizational decisions. Staff within these trusts were then officially employed by their local trust, although most remained on nationally determined terms and conditions due to the strength of their unions, which were strongly opposed to local pay (Maynard 1991). The increased autonomy for local employers allowed more flexibility for hospital management, and some used this freedom to attempt massive new change initiatives.

The development of health care reform policy in the United Kingdom involves a complex configuration of interests at the national level. The party in power has the primary ability to introduce legislation, and the British electoral system ensures that almost all the legislation originating with the government will pass.[1] All the ministers and the secretary of state are appointed by the prime minister and may be reshuffled out of the position at any time. The prime minister therefore has the power to set the policy agenda and ensure that bills are passed.

The types of reform conducted by the government can be divided into two main categories: legislated changes and regulatory changes. Regulatory changes do not necessarily require legislative approval and may include some forms of internal NHS reorganization as well as changes to the systems of audit and monitoring, which do not alter financing arrangements or governance structures. Policies that affect only terms and conditions of employment can be negotiated directly (on a tripartite basis) among the Department of Health, the NHS employers (represented by the NHS Confederation), and NHS employees (represented by more than twenty officially recognized unions). Unless the scope of the policy broadens, these regulatory changes do not need to pass through Parliament. Wider-ranging reforms, such as changes in the institutions of hospital accountability and governance, must pass through Parliament; the most recent significant example of this is the Foundation Hospitals Bill establishing a new form of quasi-autonomous NHS hospital (Department of Health 2002b).

In recent years, NHS funding has increased sometimes, particularly expenditures targeted at reducing waiting lists and addressing the shortage of nurses. The government ultimately determines the pay increase given to nurses and doctors each year, after a recommendation from the Pay Review Body, which in turn receives submissions from all the key stakeholders such as the government and the unions. Because the NHS is the largest employer in the United Kingdom, NHS wages are often constrained by the government's need to set a cautious wage pattern and to keep inflation in check.

---

1. Other MPs can introduce legislation, known as a Private Member's Bill, but these bills rarely pass.

With the notable exception of organized patient groups, the key stake-holders in health care have remained relatively stable in Britain. These organized interest groups have been forced to respond to restructuring initiatives aimed at increasing capacity and improving efficiency, frequently through the use of outsourcing and novel forms of financing and subcontracting. The restructuring of the NHS does not threaten the overarching model of a national single-payer system in which services are free at the point of use. Rather, the key reform initiatives are clustered around efforts to increase auditing and monitoring to measure (and incentivize) good performance and efforts to restructure the delivery of care to improve the patient experience while providing individualized services with better clinical outcomes. These two sets of initiatives reflect the same trends as the restructuring efforts in US hospitals.

Pay systems in the NHS have changed fairly dramatically in the last few decades. Doctors are still paid at collectively bargained rates. Other NHS staff have had nationally imposed pay levels, subject to consultation but not negotiation with the unions. These pay reforms (ultimately pay increases, although sometimes at constrained rates) have cost the NHS about £540 million (around $750 million) above the projected budget (Buchan and Evans 2007, 9). This pay reform, designed to accompany the restructuring of job roles and to more accurately reflect employee knowledge and skills, has been extremely expensive.

The most recent example of the restructuring of pay came under the Agenda for Change (AFC) project, which required the creation of new job profiles and pay for all directly employed NHS staff with the exception of doctors (Department of Health 2003a).[2] This agreement was negotiated with all the recognized NHS unions (twenty-four in total at the time) affected by the restructuring. The project entailed regrading staff according to specific skill and job profiles, rather than less accurate job titles. One impetus was the rise in pay discrimination claims that resulted from the gender stratification of the lower skilled occupations in health care. Negotiations over AFC lasted almost three years, and several unions (notably Amicus, the Society of Radiographers, and UNISON) expressed serious reservations with the final

---

2. As of this writing, this pay system is still in place.

agreement. The attempt to negotiate rather than impose change made the process much more protracted (Department of Health 2003a, 2004a; Royal College of Nursing 2003).

The evolution of AFC illustrates the difficulties of moving from policy creation into policy implementation. Although the need for some form of pay restructuring was recognized by political leaders, civil servants, and the unions, the human resources directors in the hospitals expressed deep reservations about the complexity of the new system. Much of this concern derived from the institutional memory of the previous experience of pay restructuring under the Thatcher government, which was both protracted and contentious and resulted in a system of pay and grading that was widely considered suboptimal. As one senior civil servant put it, this attempt at pay modernization "failed quite badly" (personal interview 2002). The implementation process of AFC was on a case-by-case basis, with all positions evaluated against model job profiles to determine the correct grading (and therefore pay) for any single job. Although job evaluations were supposed to be conducted in partnership between unions and hospital management, the unions also took on the role of monitors to ensure that all staff were treated fairly by their employers. Assessment of the impact of AFC has been sparse, although early findings suggest that workplace managers appreciate the new framework, while individual employees have experienced little progress (Buchan and Evans 2007). As of this writing, the AFC framework still determines pay for most NHS employees (NHS Employers 2014).

In 2003, just as the protracted AFC negotiations were reaching agreement on a new pay structure for nonmedical staff in the NHS, the government was also negotiating a new collective bargaining agreement with doctors—specifically the consultants, the 30,000 senior doctors whose professional expertise and key role in service delivery gives them leverage disproportionate to their numbers in the workforce. In 2002, a proposed consultant contract was rejected in its ratification vote by the British Medical Association. This was the first major (proposed) change to the collective bargaining agreement since the founding of the NHS in 1948. The rejected contract offered generous pay raises in return for greater managerial control over doctors. As an editorial in the *British Medical Journal* explained,

> It was rejected primarily because it gave more control to managers, people who in many hospitals are neither trusted nor respected. This might be seen

as a simple power struggle, with consultants refusing to be told what to do. Why shouldn't they get into line like most other workers?

All consultants work in teams, and most recognize that they are part of complex organizations and need to play their part. . . . Hospitals handed over entirely to managers and politicians will, consultants believe, be less responsive to patients' needs. Many managers believe the opposite. What's clear is that the NHS will not flourish unless doctors, managers, politicians, and all other staff can work well together and pursue the same goals. But perhaps this is best achieved by giving considerable autonomy to consultants. Most, after all, have done more than they are required to, even though some have abused their privileges. Consultants must accept, however, that managers play a vital role in complex organizations like health care. The beast will not run itself. (Smith 2002)

The final consultant contract, negotiated a year later, dropped many of the areas in which doctors would have ceded some control over their schedules and work organization, while retaining the generous pay increases. This affirmed the powerful role of doctors in constraining attempts at work reorganization, Maynard and Bloor argued. "Temporarily at least, the demand for clinical autonomy . . . has triumphed. At the same time, the personal income of consultants has been substantially enhanced" (Maynard and Bloor 2003, 5).

One major element of health service reform has been the growth of performance targets and indicators, particularly since the election of the Labour government in 1997. The central element of monitoring and audit of the NHS is a complex system of performance indicators. Many of the targets were informed by political considerations, in particular the Blair government's early promise to significantly reduce waiting lists for NHS treatment (Labour Party 2001). Although the targets were formulated to meet political (and electoral) objectives, the tasks of meeting and administering them fell to civil servants in the Department of Health and to health service managers in hospital workplaces. The targets are designed as both drivers and monitors of good NHS performance (personal interviews 2002). The performance indicators were nominally implemented, often in ways that produced dramatic, unintended consequences (Givan 2005).

As systems of measurement and monitoring arose in the United Kingdom, prominent scholars began to question their value. In *The Audit Society*, Michael Power (1997) argues that the culture of monitoring in the public sector is part of a larger move toward asserting centralized control. By holding local managers to so many detailed and specific standards, the government retains control over the service while still adhering to the principle of local autonomy and decentralization. Julian Le Grand (2003) argues that the imposition of greater monitoring is a symptom of a move away from regarding public service professionals as generally altruistic, possessed of a specific ethos that drives high-level performance. In the case of the NHS, local hospital trusts are told which goals they must meet, but they are (theoretically) free to determine how best to meet these goals. The dynamic of power and accountability is crucial in determining whether a policy is successfully implemented or whether local managers and frontline service providers resist or reshape the change. Where local managers feel that they have been neither consulted nor involved in the creation of the performance indicators, they are unlikely to implement them in the way intended by the original policy. As such, the government is not able to enforce policy implementation, even when it attempts to impose stiff penalties for noncompliance.

Many of the target areas in the NHS performance ratings are based on political point-scoring of the past (Hansard [Commons] 2002a, 2002b). In the United Kingdom, the opposition party traditionally has mocked the government for the length of NHS waiting lists. Unlike many aspects of health care, waiting lists are easily measurable and quantifiable. Waiting list data are easily comparable, and it is therefore fairly straightforward to track increases or decreases in the times patients wait to see a specialist doctor or the time they wait for a particular procedure. Although the Labour government successfully increased the size of the NHS workforce in order to reduce waiting lists, both new and existing staff had to embrace the "new ways of working" put forward by the government if greater efficiencies were to be realized. The waiting list targets were formulated by the government (with many of the deadlines designed with an eye to the electoral calendar), but these politicians could not ultimately determine whether the targets were met. Perversely, the pressure from the government on the workforce led to allegations of gaming the system and cheating among NHS managers (Public Administration Select Committee 2003).

The dilemma of decentralization is that if the government diffuses control, it gives up its ability to determine outcomes; but so long as the government is held politically responsible for these outcomes, it cannot completely cede control of the NHS—hence the prevalence of targets and systems of

audit. Many health service managers felt seriously constrained by the national policies and targets because these are, by nature, not sensitive to the
particularities of the local context (Givan 2005). Similarly, members of Parliament (MPs) were frustrated when hospitals were not meeting the needs
of the population they were supposed to serve. For example, one MP pointed
out that when there was no government target measuring the length of the
wait for a hip replacement, this procedure was not prioritized by the trusts
(in fact, this particular distortion of priorities was a major concern for one of
the MPs I interviewed who represented a constituency with a large elderly
population). In areas with a high proportion of elderly residents, this is a
crucial service, but trusts are unable to prioritize a service of particular local
importance such as this without failing to meet other targets and risking the
imposition of punitive measures (and without their top managers risking
unemployment due to poor performance). The system of incentives and
penalties concomitant with NHS performance ratings makes it impossible
for a trust to abandon the government's list of priorities and create its own
priorities based on local needs.

The target-setting culture that pervaded the Labour reform agenda came
under extensive criticism from the Audit Commission, a national (governmental) budget and expenditure watchdog, the House of Commons Public
Administration Select Committee, and the major health unions (Audit
Commission 2003; Public Administration Select Committee 2003). The
combined criticism from employee groups and monitoring bodies illustrates
the serious shortcomings of the target-based approach, though none of these
groups had the power to alter the procedures. The implementation of the
policy was so inconsistent that it never met its original objectives, and it has
been under constant revision by the government and its agencies ever since
(Healthcare Commission 2004). My interviews with workplace managers revealed both manipulation of data and extreme suspicion about the reliability of certain statistics (Givan 2005), so the workplace implementation of
these procedures has been a far cry from the policy as originally designed.

The NHS was originally a unitary system, with almost all services owned
and operated by the NHS itself and all staff directly employed. The only
major exception was general practitioners, who were independent contractors. In a typical hospital, however, everyone from a consultant (attending
physician) to parking attendants, maintenance staff, and technical specialists were all government employees. This employment status included

national terms and conditions of service, national pay systems, and a relatively generous government pension.

Around the mid-1980s some NHS services were subcontracted to the private sector, as Thatcher imposed competition and subcontracting across the public services (Boyne 1999). The services were similar to the work many companies subcontract, in areas such as cleaning, catering, and payroll. Since it began in the early 1990s, the use of temporary agency staff in the NHS has also increased markedly. This is especially true in nursing, where agency nurses achieve higher wages and greater flexibility in return for minimal benefits (Tailby 2005). The outsourcing of support services seems to have stabilized and stopped increasing, and there is even some evidence that providers are now in-sourcing these services, thus returning them to in-house provision by direct hospital employees (Bach, Givan, and Forth 2009).

As part of its reform agenda, the Labour government also made a commitment to diverse forms of financing of public services. This included using both private sector funding and private service providers. One of the major aspects of this reform is the Private Finance Initiative (PFI). Through PFI, private companies or consortia design, build, finance, and operate public service facilities such as schools and hospitals under a long-term (usually between twenty-five and sixty years) contract from the public sector. The main innovation in these schemes was the form of financing and the degree of control the private company had over the form of services provided. Many trade unions remain vehemently opposed to PFI on the bases that it provides inferior services and that profiting from public services is inherently wrong.

Other examples of the mixed economy of health care include the Diagnostic and Treatment Centers (akin to ambulatory clinics in the United States), many of which are operated as public–private partnerships. Similarly, to cut waiting lists in the NHS, some patients are funded to receive private treatment, either in the United Kingdom or abroad. The New Labour argument was that the market and competition should be used to provide public services where most appropriate and practical, rather than being ruled out for ideological reasons (Brown 2003). Employee groups have long argued that the growing use of private service companies to provide elements of health care is detrimental both to employees and to service users (GMB 2002a; UNISON 2002a, 2002b).

As well as subcontracting of employment, the government also adopted more sweeping programs to allow private-sector providers to operate NHS facilities at a profit. The services at these facilities remain free at the point of use, and to the patient they should be indistinguishable from any other NHS facility. The contractual arrangements at PFI hospitals and Independent Sector Treatment Centers (ISTCs) are quite complex. In the case of PFI hospitals, a private company (or usually a consortium of companies) is contracted to design, build, maintain, and operate a new hospital. The program is usually used to provide a new building for an existing, aging hospital. The company receives a long-term contract (generally thirty to fifty years) to build and manage the facility. Once the hospital is built, the private provider is responsible for the provision of the nonclinical services. The support staff are usually direct employees of the consortium, while the doctors, nurses, and other professionals remain NHS employees. The consortium receives a guaranteed annual payment for the duration of the contract.

Public sector accounting provides the main argument for PFI hospitals. By spreading the cost of a new facility over several decades rather than paying all the capital expense at once, public-sector spending does not rise dramatically in a single year. The policymakers behind PFI also argue that they are able to transfer much of the risk to the private consortium—if unexpected expenses arise, they fall to the private sector and not the public purse. As should be evident, these PFI hospitals create myriad new employment relationships that demonstrate that the NHS is no longer a unitary employer. Indeed, with the complex negotiation on behalf of support staff working in PFI facilities, those staff who were employed by the NHS are able to remain employed by the NHS, while new staff in certain jobs such as cleaning are employed by the consortium. This leads to the so-called two-tiered workforce, in which workers in the same job at the same facility may be subject to radically different pay levels and terms and conditions of employment (Bewley 2006).

Several large unions have opposed this so-called creeping privatization in principle, but in practice they have taken a more pragmatic approach. My workplace interviews revealed that private providers are not always inferior employers. In fact, strong service agreements can protect employees from budget cuts, layoffs, and work reorganization. Case study research shows that the implementation of various forms of outsourcing is highly uneven, with some contractors exploiting their employees and others essentially conforming to NHS standards of employment conditions (Bach and Givan 2010; Givan and Bach 2007).

In 2012, the Health and Social Care Act implemented by the Conservative government laid the groundwork for another cascade of changes in the UK system. This act has the potential to reshape the NHS because the power to "commission" health care has been placed in the hands of general practitioners, who vigorously fought change. Thus far, dramatic changes resulting from this act have not emerged; in fact, the effects of this act have been dwarfed by the cost pressures created by massive government cuts to the NHS. On the potential effects of the 2012 Health and Social Care Act, one report stated that "the NHS has proved to be remarkably resilient in the face of efforts by successive governments to make major changes in how it is run and there is no reason to expect things to be different this time round" (Timmins 2012).

Conclusions

Neither the US nor the UK health care system is necessarily currently at a major turning point, but they are in a process of constant change. The Health and Social Care Act of 2012 set the stage for increased private provision in the NHS but only built on the reforms of the New Labour government, which in turn had continued the process of change handed to them by the previous Conservative government (Peedell 2011). While the Conservative-led government in the United Kingdom and the Obama-led health care reform act in the United States might seem to be ushering in an era of change, this constant evolution is nothing new. Change initiatives have come to these systems from all directions and at all levels. Cost pressures in both countries have increased. While expenditures on health care have increased, so has the pressure to provide high-quality care at the lowest possible cost. In both countries, mandatory and voluntary regulators have imposed a bewildering array of standards and metrics, requiring hospitals to both change their procedures and measure their outcomes. The patient-safety movement has reached hospitals in both countries, bringing pressure to both track and reduce errors. New trends such as patient-centered care have pushed providers to reorient their work, in this case to focus clinical care around the needs and decisions of the patient rather than around organizational efficiency or physician control.

In spite of the differences in the systems in access to and payment for health care, hospitals in both countries confront similar attempts at change, often with similar outcomes. The effects of these attempts at reform reveal a decidedly mixed bag. When providers decide to flex their muscle, they are able to determine the direction of change, as illustrated by the negotiations over pay reform. There have been many changes in the past decade, however, primarily in the interest of increasing both the capacity and the quality of the health service. These changes have had a huge impact on the health service employees who must implement the changes and live with the consequences. I will demonstrate in the chapters that follow how the complex dynamics among doctors, nurses, workplace managers, and higher level decision-makers create a tangled web of interests in which change is slow and difficult and frontline health care staff play a critical role.

Chapter 3

Measuring and Rewarding Performance

Imposing Change from above in the United Kingdom

Across health care systems, the drive to monitor and improve performance is everywhere, and the United Kingdom, even with its single-payer system, is no exception. From President Obama's emphasis on cutting wasteful spending and researching comparative effectiveness, to various public and private hospital rating systems, the quest to understand, measure, and improve performance is pervasive. In both the United States and the United Kingdom, government and private entities such as the media distill various health care data into comparable information and use it to make judgments and inferences about the quality of health care available at particular hospitals and even from specific physicians. In the United States many hospitals compete directly with each other; in the United Kingdom the ratings do not necessarily attract patients but may lead directly to punishment or reward from the major regulatory bodies. In this chapter I analyze a critical case of

---

This chapter is adapted from a journal article originally published in *Personnel Review* (Givan 2005).

performance measurement and monitoring, one of the key trends seen across the Anglo-American model.

Comprehensive, comparable performance ratings were imposed on the NHS by the Blair government and first implemented in 2001. Although some measurement and incentive systems had been attempted in the previous decades, the star rating regime was novel. The previous system of performance indicators, initially developed in 1983, had not been widely disseminated to the public, nor was it used punitively by the government; these indicators were designed "to trigger enquiry rather than [to serve] as answers in themselves" (Pollitt et al. 2010, 17). In stark contrast, the star rating system, which resulted from a distillation of the performance indicators, was used to share putative performance data with the public and was the basis for both reward and punishment for hospitals and their staff (Bevan and Hood 2006). The star ratings were more definitive answers, and thus marked a turning point in government monitoring of hospitals (Pollitt et al. 2010). As one Department of Health official stated, "I don't remember any major debates on star ratings, but it was a culmination of this approach of going from indicators to measures, to incentives and targets, which we seemed to move through incredibly quickly" (Pollitt et al. 2010, 21). These incentives, and their attendant sanctions, were new and created lasting damage in the relationship between the government and frontline health care providers. This case, therefore, demonstrates the critical problems in the implementation of change without input from the front line when a new system is created for political reasons that do not align with the motivation of the frontline workers to provide high-quality patient care.

The initial star rating system encountered resistance and proved ineffective. It was dropped in 2005 and replaced with a more broad-based "annual health check," which did not create rankings or star ratings of health organizations (although newspapers were able to analyze the raw data and create their own ratings). But the legacy of the much-despised star ratings remains strong. Subsequent systems have incentivized and sanctioned performance based on these data, and have continued the process of imposing targets from above. This chapter focuses on the beginning of the current assessment regime, the creation and implementation of the star rating system, and the significant changes implemented from above with insufficient input from frontline staff and managers.

Measuring performance is never easy. The most desirable outcomes may not be easily quantifiable or measurable. Similarly, if one outcome is prioritized, another may fall by the wayside. If a hospital prioritizes a fast discharge, readmission rates may raise; if the hospital emphasizes safe staffing levels, costs may rise. In the United States, Medicare payments are beginning to be tied to performance, with the system called Hospital Value-Based Purchasing being rolled out at the time of this writing. Hospitals with poor clinical results will be punished (or incentivized) by having their payments cut, but it is not clear how the hospital will improve its performance on a lower budget. Nevertheless, accountability and incentives are the dominant trend, and market-based thinking prevails.

In the United Kingdom, performance monitoring began to dominate the lives of National Health Service (NHS) staff in the 1990s and 2000s, when it was hard to enter a hospital without experiencing eye-rolling and complaints from both management and frontline staff about the proliferation first of indicators and then of more punitive targets. The NHS is always a key issue in British elections, and in the Conservative Party's ultimately successful campaign to take power from the Labour Party in the 2010 elections, the party manifesto stated, "We can't go on with an NHS that puts targets before patients" (Conservative Party 2010). Although not entirely against targets in themselves, the Conservative Party chose to blame any problems in the NHS on the Labour government's preference for putting "targets before patients." The concern about targets and monitoring was not a minor issue affecting only patients and providers but a political hot potato closely tied to the future direction of the NHS.

When the star rating system was implemented, the NHS staff had no confidence that the performance measures captured anything real that was happening in the hospitals, and they sought ways to go around the measures without completely breaking the rules. The lack of faith in this new system, even among the top performers, may have proved fatal to it. Staff and management were more than willing to admit to me that some performance monitoring could be a good thing, but there was universal agreement that this particular system was an utter failure, brought about because it had been imposed from outside with little regard for what actually happens in hospitals.

One might think that when organizations are evaluated and ranked from best to worst, individual organizations will strive to come out on top. However, in the case of these NHS ratings, this was never the case. Commenting on the star rating system for National Health Service hospitals, one manager told me exactly how the incentive failed: "We've almost got a policy now of wanting to be in the pack. We don't want to be at the top, we don't want to be those few that are deemed to be excellent because there's only one way to go from there, and we don't want to be at the bottom" (personal interview with human resources manager, zero-star trust 2002). This example clearly demonstrates that the incentive system failed—managers were not motivated to implement the government plan because the priorities seemed so misguided. They had no reason to cooperate beyond the bare minimum or to strive for the very best rating. Rather, the managers participated in the rating system to the extent that made sense to them, considering their knowledge and experience in their own hospital. Managers took the long view that if they started off with a high rating, they could only get worse in the future. Even with this simple example, one can already tell that the ratings did not incentivize high-quality performance, as defined by those outside the hospital organization.

In recent years, health care providers and policymakers in both the United States and the United Kingdom have focused on the significant harm caused by medical errors (Department of Health 2000b, 2001a; Gordon, Mendenhall, and O'Connor 2012; Haynes et al. 2009; Kohn, Corrigan, and Donaldson 2000). Beginning about 2000, reports on the subject of medical errors received massive media and public attention in both Britain and the United States. In the report *To Err Is Human* (Kohn, Corrigan, and Donaldson 2000), the Institute of Medicine quantified both the financial cost and the annual loss of life from various forms of medical errors, from misdiagnosis to medication mistakes. The conclusion that 98,000 patients died in the United States each year from preventable errors spawned what has become known as the patient safety movement (Kohn, Corrigan, and Donaldson 2000). More recent studies have shown that this initial estimate of preventable mortality due to error was likely quite low: a more rigorous and more recent study suggested that anywhere from 200,000 to 400,000 preventable deaths per year was a more accurate range (James 2013). Proponents of patient safety tend to focus on eliminating errors, both by ensuring transparency in measuring and reporting health care processes and outcomes and by intervening in these processes. One innovation, adapted from the aviation industry, is the greater use of checklists to ensure that appropriate safety steps are always followed (Gaffney, Harden, and Seddon 2005; Gawande 2007; Gordon, Mendenhall, and O'Connor 2012; Hales and Pronovost 2006). It is clear that good record-keeping leads to good data, which can in turn help identify problems as well as the likely causes of these problems. But the questions of what to do with this data and what if any incentives to attach to it are deeply fraught.

The patient-safety movement evolved in tandem with a universal emphasis on measuring and improving quality across the health care sector (and indeed in other sectors, such as education). The push for measurement moves far beyond the reporting of errors. Rather, various public and private agencies have emphasized quantifying performance in order to track (or incentivize) improvement and to create clear comparisons among health care providers. Although I include the monitoring of errors in this chapter, this performance indicator plays a relatively small role in the overall story of a system of performance monitoring imposed from above by both elected leaders and regulators with no room for frontline input.

Research on the Star Ratings

In order to use my vertical slice approach and interview all stakeholders from the policy to the workplace level, I approached all acute, specialist, and teaching hospitals in Greater London to ask them to participate in this research. Of forty hospitals, seventeen responded positively; in each of these, I interviewed the human resources director or person in an equivalent role for forty-five to ninety minutes. Because two trusts offered two interviewees, I conducted nineteen interviews in all. Although London is not perfectly representative of the NHS, the area provides a broad range of hospitals with zero- to three-star ratings, varying staff shortage problems, and different approaches to human resource management. The participating trusts captured this diversity. I also interviewed senior civil servants in the Commission for Health Improvement and the Department of Health (primarily in the Human Resources Directorate), five in all, to provide the policy perspective on human resources ratings.

It was essential to include qualitative data derived from the interviews in this research to probe beyond the numerical performance data and understand the perceptions of the ratings as a key determinant of the use of the ratings in determining human resources strategy and to understand the effects of the indicators at the front line. The ratings data have been used and triangulated elsewhere for a more technical analysis, looking at what the data can show (see, for example, Avgar, Givan, and Liu 2011a), but in this case the original qualitative data are the key to understanding why the program, imposed from above, failed so profoundly.

Managing Performance

With more than £5 billion in new funds set aside for the NHS by the post-1997 New Labour government, the government, led by Prime Minister Tony Blair, was eager to ensure that NHS hospitals used this money responsibly. As with many areas of public spending, the government introduced a wide range of targets and assessment criteria to track the performance of the trusts. The monitoring, however, went far beyond scrutinizing how this money was spent and focused on specific policies and procedures in the hospitals, from clinical outcomes to employee absence rates. This massive performance monitoring project, however, proceeded at the same time as the supposed devolution of power to frontline staff, creating an uneasy balance of power and accountability between the center and the front line. As a 2002 report stated, "We intend to give frontline staff greater control over how local health services are delivered" (Department of Health 2002a).

As my interviews show, managers never believed that they or their staff were being granted greater autonomy. To a person, the interviewees expressed a great deal of cynicism about the new system and felt that this new form of surveillance was wasteful and counterproductive. They believed the best possible course of action was to blend in with the crowd. From the very beginning, the detailed performance monitoring made it crystal clear to managers, doctors, nurses, and support workers that they were not being given the ability to make professional decisions based on their knowledge and skills; rather, they were expected to make decisions based on priorities imposed from above. Specific performance goals were dictated from above by politicians and bureaucrats, without substantive input from anyone with real workplace experience. The lack of input into the creation of the performance standards as well as the content of the standards themselves combined to frustrate and antagonize workplace managers.

In theory, the newly introduced star rating system could have had an impact on the goals of increasing public awareness of the quality of health care provision and on improving standards of performance. In practice, however, the performance indicators never fulfilled these goals; they did not definitively improve performance, but they did create opportunities for the public to criticize rather than understand and more appropriately access the NHS. Thus, the ratings were unsuccessful because they alienated staff and created a culture of mistrust.

Although the ratings system was changed over time, it was not entirely abandoned. As of this writing, the agency responsible for the latest set of indicators, developed under a Conservative government, defensively asks and then answers on their informational web site: "Isn't this just a ranking of hospitals? No, this isn't a judgment on hospitals. The profiles [indicators] bring together information that helps us plan our inspections" (Care Quality Commission 2014a). The current monitoring agency, the Care Quality Commission, was described by one commentator as "choking on its own bile" as it continues to "acquire scalps" while controlling and redefining performance ratings, even as it admits to serious errors in its data analysis that erode any trust in the ratings by those who work in the NHS (Vize 2014).

Effective performance management in private companies or publicly owned organizations depends on the availability of accurate data that are collected in a fair and transparent way. Across the NHS no executives expressed any confidence in the quality of the data used to create the ratings. All interviewees argued that the monitoring regime created perverse incentives by emphasizing certain health conditions, ignoring others, and placing too much weight on the analysis of data that were of uneven quality at best. As one commentator wrote as recently as 2014, "The exhausting rounds of regulatory beatings are demonstrably not delivering the required change. Regulation has its place, but a narrow focus on individual organizations is the wrong approach" (Vize 2014).

In Britain during the 1980s public sector agencies were under pressure to cut costs and adopt practices previously associated with the private sector (Clarke, Gewirtz, and McLaughlin 2000, 6; McLaughlin, Osborne, and Ferlie 2002). Dawson and Dargie argued that the three priorities for public services in the 1980s became "cost containment, public support and performance improvement" (2002, 35). In performance management, the approach eventually shifted from the adoption of specific private sector management techniques to an output-focused strategy, emphasizing capacity-building and high-performance approaches, no matter where they originate. This meshed with the Blairite mantra of "what matters is what works." The Blairite agenda of public service reform adopted key elements of performance management (known by scholars and public administration professionals as "New Public Management," when brought to the public sector) while maintaining fairly strict channels of monitoring and control from the center.

Some measures of financial management were used in the NHS rating system, but the categories primarily focused on centrally defined standards of service provision, such as the rate of staff absence due to sickness, or the average waiting time for emergency room patients. This emphasis contrasted with ideals of professionalism, where a doctor or nurse can, by definition, always be trusted to perform at the highest level (Davies and Kirkpatrick 1995; Hunter 2002; Morgan and Potter 1995). Similarly, notions of a public service ethos suggested that the employees would always provide excellent service without close monitoring or additional incentives (Public Administration Select Committee 2002). Discussions of the new emphases on quality and auditing correctly argued that these new management methods are a way of asserting control (Martinez Lucio and MacKenzie 1999; Power 1997; Propper and Wilson 2003). It is not surprising, therefore, that the ratings met with a great deal of resistance from hospital trusts with both high and low star ratings because managers perceived them as a loss of local control. Stephen Bach summarized the dilemma for human resources managers: "The personnel agenda within trusts has in large part been shaped by responding to a series of frequently contradictory national policy initiatives and meeting national performance targets" (1999, 188). Managers were not given the autonomy to pursue a strategic agenda within their own hospitals.

Sandra Dawson and Charlotte Dargie described the process through which performance management could have led to service improvement: "Government ensures that good comparative performance data are collected and made public, and that consistently bad performers are identified and given support to improve; if they fail to improve they are penalized, resulting in individuals losing their jobs and/or the work undertaken by the failing organization being given to another" (2002, 50). Summarizing the objectives of the NHS performance ratings and providing a blueprint of the penalties for poor performers that the Blair government and its successors fully embraced,[1] this account does not mention the rewards that are available to high achievers. But as we will see, the notion of "good comparative performance data" was extremely contentious and thus endangered the credibility of the entire ratings system. Poor data quality was a key point of concern among trusts and between trusts and the government, causing much more consternation than the existence of the ratings themselves.

The performance ratings were one of several government initiatives designed to hold trust managers accountable for the performance of their trusts. Indeed, the star ratings held individuals (particularly chief executives) responsible for the overall performance of their organizations—those with very poor ratings could expect to lose their jobs (Carvel 2001). The heightened pressure on human resources directors to fulfill explicit objectives and achieve high ratings, along with the larger strategic role for human resources, put further strain on the ever-expanding personnel function (Bach 1999). The increase in responsibility was somewhat undermined by the increase in monitoring, as the overall policy demonstrated that the government did not have confidence in trust managers.

The ultimate reward, given to the very best three-star trusts, also showed the frustration that trust managers felt with performance management. Those trusts that were considered excellent had the opportunity to become foundation hospitals. These hospitals were given additional funding, greater autonomy, and a degree of freedom from the myriad government targets. Ironically, the reward for meeting the goals partially meant no longer having to meet all the goals. It was as if the government recognized that avoiding performance management could work as a major incentive. The NHS human resources indicators were an example of the flawed implementation of New Public Management through which local managers were essentially controlled by the central bureaucrats.

Performance indicators now pervade all aspects of health care. In human resources, indicators have evolved from raw measures of total manpower to more complex measures of human resource management, reflecting

---

1. On September 1, 2003, the management of the Good Hope Hospital Trust in Birmingham was contracted to a private sector company (Secta). The contract stated that the company must take the hospital from its present zero-star rating to three stars within three years (Shifrin 2003). This is evidence that the potential punishments for poor performance ratings were not idle threats.

the role of strategic human resource management in public service performance. The role of targets, however, remains controversial, with many public service staff unsure that ratings can drive or measure good performance.

Over recent decades there has been a general acknowledgment that human resource management can contribute to organizational performance, both in the public and private sectors, and in the workplace as well as the academic literature (Huselid 1995; Ichniowski, Shaw, and Prennushi 1997; Purcell 2004). The NHS, for example, in *HR in the NHS Plan*, stated its intent "to make clear how effective people management can really improve patient care and the patient experience" (National Workforce Taskforce, and HR Directorate 2002). The incorporation of measures of human resource management into the NHS performance indicators therefore demonstrated an acknowledgment by the government that good human resources practice can benefit the NHS more broadly (West et al. 2002). But human resources managers did not find the ratings to be either a valid indicator of human resources performance or a useful tool for improving human resource management in practice. Although human resources managers were enthusiastic about emphasizing the strategic role for human resources within the NHS, they were highly resistant to the indicators to measure their performance. They perceived them as a burden to human resources departments rather than a measure of (or incentive for) good organizational performance.

Development of Human Resources Performance Indicators in the NHS

According to Jowett and Rothwell (1988), the first known discussion of performance documentation and measurement in health care was in 1732. It was proposed by Dr. Francis Clifton, the physician to the Prince of Wales, who "first suggested that basic health care data should be gathered and used as an instrument of evaluation" (Jowett and Rothwell 1988, Table 2.1; Walker and Rosser 1993). The Lunacy Act of 1844 required hospitals to keep data on patient outcomes, categorized as dead, relieved, or unrelieved (Walker and Rosser 1993, 416). In the 1860s, the pioneering nurse Florence Nightingale also suggested that patient data should be "systematically recorded, analyzed and published to enable the work undertaken by hospitals to be assessed" (Goldacre and Griffin 1983, as quoted in Jowett and Rothwell 1988, 5). At the founding of the NHS, hospitals were not required to keep or share performance data. From the mid-1960s, NHS districts were required to keep mortality data, but these data were not necessarily compiled at the hospital level, and they were not used to evaluate or compare performance (Walker and Rosser 1993, 417). The first comprehensive performance indicators were introduced to the NHS in 1983 (after a pilot project in the northern region the year before). These initial indicators included a few basic measures of "manpower" that can be summarized into the following categories:

> Total staff numbers and (for some jobs) ratios
> Proportion of staff in each major staff group (ancillaries, nurses, doctors, etc.)
> Total staff cost
> Overtime cost
> Use of part time staff
> (Department of Health and Social Security 1983, 19; Jowett and Rothwell 1988, Table 2.2)

These indicators applied not only to the staff employed in a hospital and the cost of the staff but also to the specific ways in which the staff were used. As such, they were measures of manpower rather than human resource management. Even at this early stage, the department's report stated, "It is likely that there will be some remaining errors and inconsistencies, particularly in respect of the manpower indicators" (Department of Health and Social Security 1983, 5), perhaps foreshadowing subsequent problems with data quality.

Throughout the 1980s several groups were commissioned by the government to refine and harmonize the new rating systems (Jowett and Rothwell 1988, 9). Finally, a group was convened by the government to refine the indicators and suggest comprehensive universal indicators that could be implemented across the regional and district health authorities providing acute services. This group reported in 1987 with a set of suggested indicators, none of which addressed manpower or human resource management (Performance Indicator Group 1987, appendix 6).[2] The performance indicators

---

2. The equivalent report on indicators in community health services did recommend monitoring the number of district nurses and health visitors (Working Group on Indicators for the Community Health Services 1988).

used throughout the 1980s were widely considered to be focused primarily on cost and efficiency. The total number of indicators grew throughout the 1980s and culminated in "several hundred" indicators that were difficult for management and government to swallow (Smee 2002). From 1990 to 1997, NHS performance indicators were published annually.[3] None of the data collected covered measures of manpower or human resource management. They were focused on efficiency, waiting times, and patients' rights. The hospitals were not ranked as a result of these indicators, nor were the detailed indicators combined into a simplified index, as with the star ratings. In 1993 the government set several groups the task of simplifying and refining the existing indicators (Smee 2002, 60).

From 1997, with the election of the new Labour government, a new performance assessment framework was introduced. As Smee recounted, "The election of the Labour Government with a manifesto commitment to change the focus of performance management away from activity and efficiency and toward quality of outcome, provided the spur to develop a conceptual framework to pull together the proliferating indicator sets" (Smee 2002, 61). The new "Performance Assessment Framework" was published for consultation in 1998. The new indicators were initially implemented in 1999 and were published again in 2000. These "high-level performance indicators" did not include any measures of manpower or human resource management (NHS Executive 2000).

In 2000, the Commission for Health Improvement commenced operation and began collecting data on health service performance, emphasizing clinical governance and complementing the indicators that were gathered by the Department of Health beginning in the same year. The star ratings based on these performance indicators were first published in 2001 and continued to be published until 2005. The inclusion of measures of human resource management in these ratings was therefore a major departure from previous performance monitoring, which either ignored human resources altogether or included only a brief summary of staff numbers. This reflected the general belief that human resources practices can affect overall health service performance (see, for example, West et al. 2002).

---

3. For an example of NHS performance indicators, see https://web.archive.org/web/20091203130215/http://www.performance.doh.gov.uk/tables96.htm.

Reporting the Performance Indicators

The star ratings, from zero to three stars, incorporated a range of criteria measuring both clinical and nonclinical areas. In general, the areas measured reflected then current government targets, such as reducing waiting lists and reducing the waiting times in accident and emergency departments. They also covered general good practice, such as hospital cleanliness and timely responses to complaints. In introducing the first report of performance ratings in 2001, the Department of Health stated that "this information provides the basis for action to improve performance across the NHS" (Department of Health 2001b, 4).

The performance ratings were divided into four categories: *key targets* were given the most emphasis in calculating the overall rating of the trust; *clinical focus* covered clinical and medical performance; *capacity and capability focus* covered employment practices and data and information management (originally this category was limited to *staff focus*); and, finally, *patient focus* covered the patient experience not related to clinical factors, such as waiting lists and complaints procedures.

The categories within the NHS performance ratings system that related to staffing and human resources are outlined in Table 2. The changes in criteria over time were due to two main factors. First, the serious problems with data quality in measuring the vacancy rate led to the system's abandonment of this criterion under pressure from trust management after one year. The indicators gradually moved away from self-reported data, as allegations of cheating were widespread (Propper and Wilson 2003; Public Administration Select Committee 2003). Second, new surveys and employer obligations (such as mandatory annual appraisals for consultants) were put in place and could be measured to provide new data.

The commitment to improving the working lives of staff was one of the so-called key target areas used to give trusts a general rating, and the other measures were used to "refine the judgment" between high-performing trusts as part of the "balanced scorecard." These target areas were assigned specific criteria in order to make them measurable, and the criteria rather than the overall goals were the key points of contention. These targets used the most tangible, measurable aspects of human resources in hospitals. They did not necessarily capture all aspects of the human resources function, perhaps only the most measurable ones.

Table 2. Human resources indicators in NHS performance ratings

2000–1 Criteria	2001–2 Criteria	2002–3 Criteria	2003–4 Criteria
Commitment to improving the working lives of staff (key target)	Commitment to improving the working lives of staff (key target)	Commitment to improving the working lives of staff (key target)	Commitment to improving the working lives of staff (key target). Improving working lives was removed from the key targets for the 2004–5 ratings (Commission for Health Improvement 2004).
Compliance with the "New deal on junior doctors' hours" (working a maximum 56-hour week)	Compliance with the New Deal on junior doctors' hours (56-hour week)	Compliance with the New Deal on junior doctors' hours (56-hour week)	Compliance with the New Deal on junior doctors' hours (56-hour week)
Sickness/absence rate for directly employed NHS staff	Sickness/absence rate for directly employed NHS staff	Sickness/absence rate for directly employed NHS staff	
The rates of vacancies for the following key staff groups (measured as vacancies lasting three or more months): • consultants; • qualified nurses, midwives, and health visitors; • qualified allied health professionals.			
	Response to staff opinion survey on employee satisfaction with employer	Response to staff opinion survey on employee satisfaction with employer	Response to staff opinion survey on employee satisfaction with employer (renamed "staff attitudes")

(continued)

Table 2. Human resources indicators in NHS performance ratings *(continued)*

2000–1 Criteria	2001–2 Criteria	2002–3 Criteria	2003–4 Criteria
		Consultant appraisal (percentage of consultants who have completed annual appraisal)	Consultant appraisal (percentage of consultants who have completed annual appraisal and have a personal development plan)
			Health, safety, and incidents (from staff opinion survey)
			Human resource management (from staff opinion survey). For all three 2003–4 indicators using the staff survey, the precise form of the indicator was not released by the Healthcare Commission. The use of composite indicators may have provoked controversy about the relative weight given to different factors.

Sources: Department of Health 2001, 2002c; Commission for Health Improvement 2003b; Healthcare Commission 2004.

Perceptions of the Human Resources Indicators

My interviews revealed that the star rating system suffered from a serious lack of confidence and credibility: "There are trusts I know have a high star rating that I wouldn't touch with a ten foot barge pole" (personal interview with trust manager, one-star trust 2002). Liam Fox, the Shadow Health Secretary, claimed, "The star ratings system is ludicrous and should be scrapped. The ratings bear no relation to the quality of care that patients are receiving" (2003, quoted in Carvel 2003).

There was absolute consensus among human resources directors that the indicators in their current form were neither accurate nor effective because they both measured the wrong outcomes and collected poor-quality data on those outcomes. There was general unanimity that the star ratings did not provide any benefit to human resources departments in hospital trusts nor did they drive improved performance. The ratings were universally perceived as a burden. This was true across trusts, regardless of the overall or human resources–related ratings they were awarded. Only two human resources directors argued that reformulated ratings might be useful to their departments. My questions on the impact, usefulness, or accuracy of star ratings were often greeted with sarcastic laughter. One human resources director in a two-star trust described the ratings as "completely irrelevant to human resources," in spite of the prominence of measures pertaining directly to staffing issues. Another, in a one-star trust, said, "It's a pretty pointless bloody system."

James Strachan, the chairman of the Audit Commission, argued before the Public Affairs Select Committee that "there is still a real paucity at the senior level of people who are involved in the setting of targets, a lack of real world delivery experience" (Public Administration Select Committee 2003, sect. 38). Human resources directors perceived a gap between the objectives of the targets and the reality of service delivery, even among those policymakers with frontline NHS experience. As one argued, "You sometimes wonder . . . about the memory of the people making the national policy, because most of them have worked in the NHS, . . . on the shop floor, in a trust, and . . . they make suggestions that make you wonder if they've ever worked in the NHS, never mind in a hospital" (personal interview with trust manager, two-star trust, 2002).

The specific indicators relating to human resources ideally would have presented an overall assessment of how well the hospital fulfilled the human resources function as a key element of overall trust performance. But the criteria for improving working lives and the New Deal for junior doctors simply assessed whether the trust had complied with earlier initiatives.[4]

---

4. In the case of the improving working lives criterion, all trusts in the 2000–1 report were already complying with this standard (having attained pledge status within the initiative). It

The improving working lives standard was a set of human resources–related practices introduced in 2000; it required employers to implement a number of policies, from flexible working hours and retirement to child care options and professional development, in order to improve the lives of their staff and reduce burnout and attrition (Department of Health 2000a, 2003b). The New Deal for junior doctors was an initiative to cut down on the excessive and dangerous working hours of house staff and to regulate the number of hours they could work. This standard essentially used the ratings as a monitoring device rather than an incentive for further improvement; a consultation document suggested that the ratings should be explicitly divided into core standards and developmental (aspirational) standards (Department of Health 2004b). This would have potentially separated the ratings into categories of basic regulatory compliance and measures of performance above and beyond minimum acceptable standards. The sickness/absence rate assessed the percentage of staff who were absent on the average day, a widely accepted measure of human resources performance and a simple way to monitor improvement; however, this rating was dropped fairly quickly. The Department of Health was unwilling to give a specific reason for this change, but poor data quality and inaccurate self-reporting are the likely explanations.

The vacancy rate, used in 2000–2001 but abandoned by 2001–2, was highly controversial. Human resources directors uniformly spoke with distrust of this measure, and their attitudes ranged from anger to derision. All felt that the three-month vacancy rate was not useful. Most interviewees reported that they did not keep this kind of data, so they were forced to guess or estimate when submitting the numbers to the Department of Health. The three-month vacancy rate was described as "total rubbish" and "complete nonsense," with the assertion that "people make [the numbers] up," by human resources directors in two-star and three-star trusts. The Public

---

therefore did not provide any means for differentiating between trusts, and it is unclear whether the Performance Ratings themselves provided any further incentive for compliance. In contrast, although the vast majority of trusts achieved compliance with the New Deal for junior doctors' hours, a significant number of trusts "underachieved" and "significantly underachieved," thus showing that the target was probably more meaningful. One would expect that the money and emphasis put into this particular initiative would mean that compliance rates would increase dramatically and that its universal implementation might eventually render it redundant as a performance criterion.

Administration Select Committee confirmed this notion, stating that "allegations of cheating, perverse consequences and distortions in pursuit of targets, along with unfair pressure on professionals, continue to appear" (Public Administration Select Committee 2003, sect. 28).

My interviews revealed that the distrust of this rating threw other ratings into question, making it much more difficult to convince managers of the value of any of the performance indicators. It is clear that this distrust has remained as the performance regime has evolved over successive governments. In 2014, one prominent commentator wrote that "at present the overriding objective for any NHS organization is to avoid being picked up by the regulators' radar. Managers know that, like some piece of high-tech weaponry, once a regulator is locked on to you it is perilously difficult to shake them off" (Vize 2014).

This lack of confidence suggested that conclusions drawn on the basis of these indicators may have been disregarded by the same professionals who were supposed to benefit from this performance review. Ultimately, the Department of Health discontinued the use of the vacancy statistic, regarding it as "unhelpful" and "a potential disincentive," according to a senior civil servant.

As data quality in trusts improved, for example, through the Electronic Staff Record, vacancy rates and total staff numbers (including nurse/patient ratios) returned to the overall performance ratings; this would satisfy the condition, suggested by Carol Propper and Deborah Wilson, that there be "non-corruptible indicators of performance . . . not subject to manipulation by the individuals whose actions are being measured" (2003, 265). The increased weight given to indicators derived from staff surveys rather than from the self-reporting of managers was another move away from corruptible measures. Also, the inclusion of specific measures of data quality and information management may have increased confidence in some ratings.

Many human resources directors recognized that the prominence of staffing concerns in the overall ratings was the first major acknowledgment by the government that human resources factors represented a significant component of positive trust performance. Human resources directors overwhelmingly embraced this development. One spoke of human resources having more "clout" in the overall management of the trust. Another spoke of being able to fund important initiatives without having to convince the trust's financial managers that they were essential. Although many were critical of the specifics of the criteria and statistics used, they were very pleased that their area of responsibility was being given such prominence. Many felt that this prod from the government had forced trust boards and executives to place new emphasis on staffing issues, an area that had often been overlooked in the past. Perhaps this experience revealed to them that it might possible to measure human resources performance in a way that was more acceptable and useful to human resources managers. Perhaps it also impressed on them how poor quality data can wholly undermine a potential driver of good human resources performance. There is a paradox here: these human resources directors claimed that they would like more clout and acknowledgment, but at the same time they expressed deep hostility toward these specific ratings. Given that the ratings were perceived as only punitive, with no sense of positive reinforcement or developmental emphasis, it is perhaps unsurprising that managers were deeply dissatisfied with them.

Human resources directors were concerned that areas that were excluded from performance ratings—from health conditions that were ignored, to professional development opportunities—would ultimately be neglected. It is impractical (or rather, impossible) to rate a trust on every aspect of its work, but when certain targets are emphasized, nontarget areas are likely to be deemphasized. One human resources director in a two-star trust stated that "the issues that are measured for the star ratings, we push on" and added that "there are probably other things as well that are, to me, more important that don't get the push" (personal interview 2002). These areas might have included training and staff development, and retention initiatives responsive to specific needs of the staff in a specific community, who might have particular challenges in areas such as high housing costs or a need for on-site childcare. When trusts are unable to set their own priorities, they lose autonomy, without regard for any local factors that might make different targets more appropriate. The trusts' lack of input into priorities ran counter to the government's claim of devolving decision-making power to frontline staff.

Other instances of manipulation of priorities included the performance indicators for consultant appraisal as well as for treatment of specific medical conditions (such as fractured hips and breast cancer). According to one group of scholars (who compared the manipulation of NHS data to the gaming of the system by bureaucrats that was rampant in the Soviet Union), "There was no systematic audit of the extent to which the reported successes in English health care performance . . . were undermined by gaming and measurement problems, even though much of the data came from the institutions who were rated on the basis of the information they provided" (Bevan and Hood 2006, 530).

Managers tended to trust the ratings when they felt that they had been consulted over the most appropriate rating criteria; for example, they felt that the improving working lives standard, which reflected the implementation of a wide-ranging and well-liked set of initiatives, was appropriate and relevant. Many human resources directors stated that they had expressed their dissatisfaction with the use of the vacancy rate as a performance criterion. Responses were mixed on whether policymakers listen to the opinions of practitioners. Although one manager said, "We are managing to input to the center what we think are the real indicators of human resources performance," no managers felt that the government was responsive to their concerns. The overall perceived lack of consultation was a key problem for managers, and this perception reinforced their doubts about the usefulness of the ratings. For example, two different interviewees emphasized the absence of consultation:

> We do influence things but a number of things just emerge without any consultation and we're told what to do.

> I wouldn't say we're ever consulted adequately over changes in national policy, but to some extent if you work in the public sector you don't always expect to be consulted on policy, you know the vision is going to be somebody else's. What has happened over the last two to three years is not only is the vision somebody else's but we're actually prescribed in very great detail how to implement that vision, which is irksome. (Personal interview with human resources manager, two-star trust, 2002)

This concern about the process of implementation was really a concern with the imposition of priorities from above; for example, government agencies proclaimed that the vacancy rate in itself was a problem, rather than allowing local managers to develop locally appropriate policies to improve recruitment and retention. In theory, one could reduce the vacancy rate by relying on temporary agency workers and the hiring of staff who are unlikely to commit to the organization for a long period of time. Local human resources directors expressed a strong desire to address broad problems by using their locally honed expertise, rather than simply trying to address one minor aspect of the bigger problem in order to avoid punishment for failing to meet a target.

Consequences of the Human Resources Indicators

One might assume that this rating system would be a simultaneous carrot and stick that rewarded high-performing trusts with acclaim, further autonomy, and financial incentives and that punished those that were deemed below par. But managers felt that the stick was much stronger than the carrot. Most stated that the advantages of being a three-star trust paled in comparison with the disadvantages of being a zero-star trust. Some also felt that being awarded three stars was something of a mixed blessing.

Almost all those interviewed spoke specifically of the problems of trusts awarded no stars in the performance ratings. In particular, staff recruitment and morale problems were highlighted. Within the current labor market, with staff shortages in many key areas, staff have a good deal of choice about where to work. In an area like London, with its large number of hospitals, often in close proximity to each other, recruitment problems were only exacerbated by a zero-star rating. One human resources director said of trusts with a poor star rating:

> Do I think that people will be demoralized if they hear their trust gets one star? Yes, I definitely do, I think they'll be demoralized on two counts. Firstly, I think it will confirm every negative feeling they've ever had about the trust and secondly I think, particularly for nursing staff, for all health care staff at the moment, everyone is working to do two people's jobs, in my opinion. It is grueling. It's particularly grueling out on the wards. I believe that the biggest motivator for a nurse . . . is a desire to give at least adequate if not good patient care. . . . And so when they are running so fast to try and achieve that and they hear their trust has got a one star rating it . . . must really hurt at a very personal level I suspect, [they will say] "I just can't do this anymore." (Personal interview with human resources manager, one-star trust, 2002)

Rather than encouraging low-rated trusts to learn from their peers and improve their performance, the ratings sometimes served to reinforce existing concerns, lower general morale, and make the task of improvement even more difficult. Another human resources director (in a two-star trust) stated that star ratings "make a difference to me because nobody wants to work in a no-star trust because you get your head chopped off." Significantly, the overall rating of a trust, not just its human resources score, is likely to have an impact on staff and staffing issues within the trust. Department of Health officials, while sympathetic to this concern (especially as it might affect recruitment), felt that it was ultimately more important to identify underperforming trusts and encourage them to improve. One senior civil servant stated that "a year of bitter medicine is probably worth taking if it turns around a situation that has been stuck forever" (personal interview, 2002). In other words, something had to be done. But with this deep animosity toward the ratings, there is little evidence that situations were turned around.

The incentives for high-performing trusts were also somewhat perverse. Human resources directors at two trusts with two stars spoke specifically of their preference for being given two, rather than three stars. Both felt that they would be uncomfortable with the notion that they could only go down, rather than up the performance ladder. One human resources director described his trust as being "highly delighted" to be given a two-star ratings, as it showed "there's still something to achieve, and we aren't crap" (personal interview, 2002). In this instance, the awarding of three stars was not necessarily an objective for a trust, which again raised the question about the performance ratings as a positive incentive.

Performance Management Today

When the star ratings were abandoned in 2005, the Healthcare Commission reformulated the ratings and eliminated the distillation of the metrics into a single rating. From 2005 to 2009, the Healthcare Commission used an "annual health check," which rated the hospital on similar criteria to those used under the previous system but also included an inspection of each hospital. In 2009, the rating system was modified again, and with the election of the Conservative-Liberal coalition government in 2010, the ratings changed yet again (with the Conservatives stating that their priority was sharing detailed data with patients). Indeed, within a few weeks of coming into office, the coalition government began to publish weekly reports of Methicillin-resistant *Staphylococcus aureus* (MRSA) and *Clostridium difficile* (C.diff) infection rates in hospitals. A series of different regulators was given responsibility for administering the system, and in an attempt to demonstrate the ways in which it was substantively improving health care system performance, each new government and health secretary modified the specific indicators used (Nuffield Trust 2013). Although the ratings have continued to evolve, the regime of targets and incentives remains in place.

The ratings established in 2014 look at many more health conditions and performance areas. There is a focus on "outliers" in performance rate—in other words, the analysis emphasizes areas in which a hospital's mortality rates are significantly higher than those of other hospitals for a specific department or group of health conditions. But so long as being an "outlier" results in punishment rather than developmental assistance, financial investment, or any true assistance with improvement, the monitoring regime remains deeply punitive and subject to manipulation by those responsible for reporting the data. Any hospital hoping for a positive rating will place resources (both human and financial) into the areas that are measured, and with both money and staff in short supply, other areas are likely to suffer.

Clearly, it would be impossible to set ambitious and achievable targets for every aspect of good human resources practice or every medical condition. Nevertheless, because the performance indicators do determine the strategic emphasis of trust managers, if they are going to improve performance the indicators must be appropriate and perceived as such. As one human resources director said, "You should always be pushing on [staff] sickness, you should always have programs of staff involvement, but there are probably other things as well that are, to me, more important that don't get the push, like training and development programs. Nobody star rates you on those and I actually think they're critical" (personal interview with human resources manager, two-star trust, 2002). Training and development only began to be measured several years after the star rating system began.

The very existence of the ratings makes those in many trusts feel that they are being monitored with constant suspicion. Michael Power (1997) argues that this type of performance auditing stems from a lack of trust between agencies. The mutual distrust that emerges from the ratings system is unlikely to foster positive relationships among managers, staff, and patients in the National Health Service. The problems with self-reported data have only reinforced this suspicion and distrust. Ultimately, this leads to a lack of respect for the ratings and the degrading of any positive incentives that could result from them.

As the ideology underpinning the ratings regime has remained relatively intact, a new approach has been proposed by some NHS providers, working thus far outside the performance rating regime of the Care Quality Commission. These NHS providers have taken it upon themselves to work collaboratively to improve health care quality without assuming the role of punishers. One observer described this novel approach as "solutions-focused systems reform" by which "the role of the regulators . . . would be to facilitate ground-up reform by removing barriers and changing the flows of money to promote the growth of community provision, break down the artificial divide between primary and secondary care and emphasize population health and prevention" (Vize 2014).

According to the Audit Commission, a performance measurement system should have the following attributes: clarity of purpose, focus, alignment (with larger goals), balance, regular refinement, and robust performance indicators (Audit Commission 2000). In the case of the star rating system, the human resources performance indicators never met the criteria of robustness. In a separate report, the Audit Commission also claimed that "initial staff resistance to gathering performance data can be overcome if staff believe that the information is going to be useful to them as well as to others" (Audit Commission 1999). None of my interviewees saw any benefit to themselves as human resources managers in the practice of performance indicators, and this made the ratings more of a bureaucratic burden than a driver of positive change. A more collaborative approach, with a focus on development rather than punishment, would likely increase the buy-in from hospital managers.

Propper and Wilson ask the question "Do PMs [performance measures] help agencies achieve the goals they have been set by policy-makers?" (2003, 251). The answer in the star rating case seems to be no. The indicators neither appropriately measured nor incentivized the government's targets for human resource management in the NHS.

One point that has not been addressed in the literature is that the ranking nature of the star ratings may have been one of its key drawbacks. With the government emphasizing that a balanced approach is crucial and the star ratings, rather than the detailed indicators, being the cause of low morale, it becomes unclear whether distilling the indicators into simplified star ratings could provide anything beneficial. With refinement of the indicators, however, it may be possible to collect high-quality data that effectively measure human resources performance. For example, automated systems now make it possible for the Care Quality Commission to extract staffing data directly from a computer system rather than relying on numbers reported by managers in a survey.

Nevertheless, the ratings have an uphill battle to overcome the initial problems with the system and become useful. The managers did not see any benefit to their trusts from the performance indicators. Unless this changes, it is unlikely that the indicators can drive performance, even if they are eventually able to measure performance accurately. Even with the Cameron government's commitment to changing the indicators, the same problems persist. Sure enough, although the ratings and administering agencies have all changed names, there is now a new set of ratings administered by the Care Quality Commission with which hospitals must concern themselves, similarly created with no input from frontline workers. The ratings, known as Intelligent Monitoring, collect more than one hundred and twenty-five points of data from hospitals to determine the level of risk at which a hospital is operating (Care Quality Commission 2014a, 2014b).

Some scholars continue to argue that targets drive performance improvement (Connolly, Bevan, and Mays 2010), but these arguments quickly become tautological and return to the questions of what should be measured and how. The human resources and employee-related measures in the latest system (as of this writing) are based on more objective data extracted from electronic staff records; they include sickness rates, turnover rates, distribution ratios of staff across skill and experience (senior to junior doctors, registered nurses to other staff, high-level registered nurses to other registered nurses, etc.). The indicators also include criteria obtained from staff surveys on areas such as whether an employee would recommend his or her hospital as a place to work or receive treatment, and whether staff have access to training or appraisal (Care Quality Commission 2014b). Onsite inspectors are also supposed to assess whether both job training and staff supervision are effective (Care Quality Commission 2014a). As of June 2014, the government also had created a public-facing web site with data on all hospitals, emphasizing patient safety (as measured by indicators such as appropriate staffing levels and honest, transparent reporting of problems).

In a sense, this system has a lot in common with the detested star ratings. Each hospital is graded in crude categories that lack nuance—green for good, blue for OK, and red for poor (NHS Choices 2015—and the use of standard definitions to create supposedly objective data has remained contentious and difficult to achieve (Audit Commission 2012). The new measures emphasize prevention of patient falls and pressure sores while, for example, ignoring urinary tract infections that can result from the careless use of catheters. The government and regulators have apparently learned few lessons over the last decade, and the system has come full circle. It is not hard to imagine the results that these new crude measures might produce. One can expect the gamut of outcomes that were seen in the previous rounds of hospital ratings, from data manipulation and lying, to the neglect of any hospital activity that is not emphasized in a government performance indicator.

Closing Observations

It is not fair to say that no rating system would or could ever work. Rather, one can identify problems with the practical application of such systems. The first problem is data quality. Whether through intentional distortion or manipulation, sloppy record keeping, or simple human error, the data used to monitor and rate hospitals are often of substandard quality. Some rating systems use survey data (often from patients, sometimes from staff) that can improve the quality tremendously and increase the sample size. Surveys can measure what a hospital is actually doing, rather than what its management claims it is doing.

Ratings systems that rely on clinical outcomes as reported by hospital management are never likely to achieve a high degree of credibility. Some hospitals monitor their own progress, particularly in using data from their own digital systems, and many have used this self-monitoring to drive self-improvement. This was the case in Maimonides hospital in Brooklyn, New York, when the hospital dramatically improved its speed in responding to bedside alarms, as discussed in chapter 6. In general, however, outside monitors face an uphill task in gaining the trust of hospitals. Even surprise inspections or the use of data originally collected for other purposes is often insufficient to make hospital management and staff confident that these measures actually report the quality of the hospital in a useful way.

So long as the data are of poor quality or are even perceived to be poor quality, these ratings will never be fully credible. Perhaps the best fix is to remove punitive ratings from the equation, and instead, in an effort led by those in the hospitals with the greatest understanding of the current challenges, to emphasize a collaborative approach that allows for the sharing of best practices and the allocation of money toward investment and improvement (Vize 2014).

The second major drawback of performance monitoring is that it skews hospital priorities in inappropriate ways. Just as teachers are often accused of teaching to the test, hospitals may be accused of emphasizing the areas and conditions on which they are being rated, to the detriment of other areas. For example, if hospitals are compared on the basis of their outcomes for heart attack patients but not stroke patients, it is only logical that the hospital may put more resources into the treatment of heart attacks. This is especially true when something material is at stake—whether it is the job of a hospital executive or a coveted position in a ranking index. As one commentator in the *British Medical Journal* put it, "The preoccupation with hitting targets results in the actual journey an individual patient experiences becoming secondary; performance is determined against crude indicators, not the expectations and experience of those using the service" (Gubb 2009). Even if the data quality is excellent, if hospital staff believe the wrong things are being measured, the ratings not only lose credibility but may also distort priorities and ultimately damage patient care by weakening staff morale and leading to more problems with recruitment and retention, which ultimately creates more challenges to high-quality patient care.

Chapter 4

REGULATING THE FRONT LINE FROM ABOVE

The Joint Commission and Hospital Regulation in the United States

Although the casual observer may see that the American health care system is fragmented and market driven, the underlying reality is that it is also highly regulated. Just as in the United Kingdom, in the United States there is a complex, overlapping web of regulating agencies that make crucial decisions in perpetuating the status quo, promulgating change, and incentivizing certain activities and priorities. These agencies, some governmental, some nongovernmental, work outside and above the health care providers (and insurers), and when they initiate change, they do so from above. Regulation serves a number of purposes, from protecting patients to preventing fraud. Regulatory agencies and licensing bodies control all health care systems and affect a wide range of functions, from laws regarding drug and device approval to the credentialing of physicians and nurses, to building codes, accounting laws, and so on.

Centralization of regulation is another key trend that affects hospitals across the Anglo-American model. There is no a priori reason why these regulatory bodies cannot be responsive to changes suggested or initiated by frontline workers (as described in the case of needlestick safety in chapter 6), but for the most part these organizations rely on their own professional expertise to nudge hospitals into particular practices.

Both the status quo and any change in health care delivery are regulated by someone or something. In the United Kingdom these regulators tend to be national agencies, headed by government-appointed officials and funded by the government, from the agencies responsible to professional licensing for health care providers, to the National Institute for Clinical Excellence (NICE), which approves or rejects medication and treatment protocols. In the United States, regulation is far more complex. The regulators are a patchwork of public and private (usually nonprofit) entities that control the health care market. Essentially these entities determine who can and cannot offer health care. As one newspaper report on the oversight system put it, "unlike some other nations . . . the United States has no federal agency charged with hospital oversight. Instead, it relies on a patchwork of state health departments and a nonprofit group called the Joint Commission that sets basic quality standards for the nation. Hospitals are rarely closed or hit with significant financial penalties for hurting patients" (Berenson 2008). One scholar describes government regulation of health care quality in the United States as "minimal" (Michael 1995, 610). The regulators in this patchwork are dominated by physicians who have become professional regulators (although to be sure, some still practice in one capacity or another).

Adding further complexity to the US picture is the fact that the health insurance industry operates under an entirely different set of rules and regulations than the health care providers. It is governed by state law and usually monitored by state insurance commissioners. One might imagine a market-driven system of health care provision, but in fact this sector is controlled by a complex set of both requirements and government practices that mean hospitals operate under what is essentially a unified, national regulatory system rather than a fragmented state-level or market-driven system.

In this chapter I examine the role of the US regulators in promulgating change by focusing on the case of Joint Commission accreditation (the Joint Commission formerly operated under several variations of this name and is perhaps still most well known as JCAHO, the Joint Commission for the Accreditation of Hospital Organizations). Like the star rating system in the United Kingdom, this case of regulation in the United States demonstrates the difficulty of implementing change in hospitals when that change comes from outside the hospital organization, and particularly when that change is neither wanted nor accepted by the managers and staff responsible for its execution.

Crucially, the Joint Commission is theoretically a voluntary organization, but in practice hospitals in the United States cannot function without the approval of the Joint Commission, as both government health care programs and private health insurers will reimburse only Joint Commission–approved health care providers. Equally significant, though, is that "the commission lacks the heft and enforcement powers of a federal regulator" (Berenson 2008). In this sense, the Joint Commission is a privatized regulator with all carrots and no sticks. As one scholar stated the case, "Though participation in the Joint Commission hospital accreditation program is still in theory voluntary, it would be very difficult for a sizeable hospital to forgo accreditation" (Jost 1994, 32). Indeed, a group of authors including the president of the Joint Commission referred to the combined Joint Commission and Centers for Medicare and Medicaid Services (CMS) regime as "national quality programs" in an analysis of performance and quality monitoring systems (Chassin et al. 2010).

States retain a great deal of responsibility for health care regulation, and "most states don't bother to inspect [Joint Commission] accredited hospitals for health or safety problems; they simply consider these hospitals as good as licensed" (Abramowitz 1991). The role of the commission has generally been beneficial (and arguably efficient) for health care providers, government and private health care purchasers (such as Medicare/Medicaid and insurance companies), and state regulators because it creates a unified regulatory framework rather than a varied and uncoordinated patchwork of accreditation standards. As one high-level official at the Joint Commission put it to me as an example, "Organizations whether they're accredited or not tend to abide by the National Patient Safety Goals, so the nation has adopted this" (personal interview 2014). This efficient solution is essentially a unified national regulatory structure controlled by a private organization rather than a public entity.

The force of the voluntary, in name but not in practice, accreditation system ruled by the Joint Commission combines with the Conditions of Participation in Medicare and Medicaid to make the reality a system of national regulation. But unlike in the United Kingdom where the regulators are government agencies, the provider-led accreditation system under the Joint Commission leaves health care providers, especially physicians, with a tremendous amount of power over the protocols and priorities of frontline health care providers. A Joint Commission leader whom I interviewed insisted to me that the commission is "physician-led" rather than "physician-dominated" (personal interview 2014). However, with the leadership of physicians and the corporate membership in the commission of the American Hospital Association, the American Medical Association, the American College of Physicians, the American College of Surgeons, and the American Dental Association, it is clear that the commission is dominated by the interests of providers, with an emphasis on physicians and not the other professional groups (Joint Commission 2012b).

Given the powerful regulation from above, change almost always emanates from above, whether through patient-safety initiatives, strongly promoted by the Joint Commission, or through payment reform by the CMS that profoundly affects the ways in which clinicians can deliver health care by controlling the reimbursement process. The power lies with the status quo and the top-down regulators, who can try to propagate change without a deep connection to those on the front lines of health care; instead, they have an abundance of input from doctors and a distinct lack of input from any other participants in the hospital team.

The combination of the lack of a direct government health care regulator and the extreme unlikelihood of health care providers losing Joint Commission accreditation has riled some critics (Jost 1983, 1994). Some have focused on the lack of government control of the commission, while others have examined the power structures and professional and industry control within the commission itself. The federal system means that states govern some aspects of health regulation, such as professional licensing, while the federal government governs others, such as drug and device approval, and independent organizations control still others. Moncrieff and Lee (2012) discuss the "functional federalism" of health care regulation in a prescriptive article suggesting that the government should promulgate national regulations that are flexible enough to respond to state-level needs and concerns. This would allow the regulators to benefit from economies of scale while potentially maintaining the degree of state control that is often necessary in the contemporary US political environment.

A Brief History of Provider-Led Regulation

In the United Kingdom, the regulation of health service has been the responsibility of the government, which is both the payer and the provider, but in the United States the providers (specifically physicians and hospitals) have taken on the lead role. In the United Kingdom, the regulators have some distance from the providers, and the professional associations and organizations of NHS managers have little influence, sometimes much to their chagrin. In the United States, this regulation, particularly the promulgation and enforcement of uniform standards, is instituted by the providers themselves and then accepted by the payers, both the government and insurance companies. It is worth noting that these most privileged providers do not represent all providers, as nonphysicians are sparsely represented, and large hospital groups and health care systems dominate the main regulatory body. The organizational structure of the Joint Commission might lead to accusations of vampires guarding the blood bank, but in fact my research showed that most hospital administrators and managers (including physician managers) do not feel at all connected to the commission: they view it as a threatening outsider rather than as a cozy self-regulator.

The first precursor to the Joint Commission was a brief set of rules, the Minimum Standard adopted by the American College of Surgeons (ACS) in 1919. These rules were intended to require certain things of hospitals where ACS members practiced. The single page of requirements stated, in summary, that:

1. All doctors practicing in the hospital be defined as "staff."
2. Only well-qualified, licensed physicians should be allowed to be "staff."
3. Staff govern "the professional rules of the hospital."
4. "Accurate and meticulous records [should] be written for all patients."
5. "Diagnostic and therapeutic facilities" should include at least a clinical laboratory and an X-ray department. (American College of Surgeons 1919)

It is not clear what recourse was available for noncompliance with this voluntary standard or whether ACS members would refuse to practice at hospitals that were out of compliance. It is important to note that many of these requirements are paradigmatic examples of professionals exerting control over both their work and the membership of their profession (essentially the labor supply). The fact that these requirements fit on a single page has today become a recurring joke for administrators and medical professionals, who are accustomed to the endless paperwork of the current Joint Commission requirements. These early regulations that began with exerting control over professionals and the hospitals employing them have evolved into rules that more directly ensure high-quality patient care.

The organization now known as the Joint Commission was created in 1951 as "an independent, not-for-profit organization . . . whose primary purpose is voluntary accreditation" (Joint Commission 2012b). The members of the Joint Commission on Accreditation of Hospitals, as it was then called, were corporate members—organizations with a strong interest in creating universal quality standards in hospitals: the American College of Surgeons (which already administered a voluntary inspection system for hospitals), the American College of Physicians, the American Hospital Association, the American Medical Association, and the Canadian Medical Association. This was a powerful coalition of health care providers, with no representation from those without a vested financial interest in controlling the health care market (either the labor market or delivery itself).

As with much US health care, the 1960s marked a key turning point for the commission. Not only did the rise of the health maintenance organization (HMO) occur in the 1960s (and then again the 1990s), but the creation of Medicare and Medicaid brought massive changes to the health care industry. Critically, in heavily privileging the role of the commission (then called the Joint Commission for the Accreditation of Hospitals, or JCAH), the Social Security Amendments passed by Congress in 1965 awarded this deeming power to the JCAH (Joint Commission 2012b). Essentially, any hospital that was accredited by the JCAH was deemed to be compliant with Medicare regulations and therefore eligible to serve these patients and access this massive new revenue stream. This power was established when Medicare was created, and the commission has held this privileged role throughout Medicare's lifetime.

At this point, it is fair to say that the JCAH began functioning as a government regulator, even while retaining its operational independence. Indeed, in the early days of Medicare, the JCAH was not obligated to share any of the details of its accreditation reviews with the government department responsible for Medicare and Medicaid (the Department of Health, Education and Welfare). More transparency was eventually legislated and expanded in 1970s after consumer pressure and some Freedom of Information Act requests (Jost 1994, 19). In the decades since then, the CMS has expanded the deeming authority of the Joint Commission, and the commission has no real national competitor in its business of accreditation, although some states do retain their own accreditation system for Medicaid.

The Joint Commission initially based its accreditation on hospitals' practices and procedures rather than on clinical or performance outcomes. For example, the accreditors would ask whether there were systems in place for examining clinical outcomes, rather than requesting data on the outcomes themselves (Ratcliffe 2009, 316). In New York State in the mid-1980s, there were a number of serious and possibly preventable incidents in hospitals that had Joint Commission accreditation, and several studies and commissions began to examine whether the Joint Commission was accrediting hospitals that were offering substandard care (Ratcliffe 2009). In response to some very public criticism, the commission began to rework its ratings system under a program called Agenda for Change, which moved some of the accreditation process into the examination of outcomes and performance rather than policies and structures.[1]

By the late 1990s, some politicians were questioning whether JCAHO had unchecked or inappropriate power in the regulation and provision of health care. The key questions were whether the commission was accountable to the government and whether the government (specifically the CMS) had delegated important powers of accreditation to an unregulated, unaccountable, and autonomous organization that could shape health care provision according to its own whims or according to the narrow interests of physicians, who dominated the organization. In 1998, Congressman Pete Stark (who would lead the drive to put JCAHO on a level playing field a decade later) submitted extended remarks on the role of the commission to the *Congressional Record*. His comments began with a basic point on accountability: "We need to take immediate action to make JCAHO accountable to the public." He went on to detail the reasons behind his (at that point)

---

1. The Joint Commission's Agenda for Change had nothing to do with the health care worker pay restructuring in the United Kingdom in the 1990s that went by the same name.

eight-year battle for increased accountability to both the federal government and the public (Stark 1998).

Stark was particularly concerned about the conflict of interest inherent in the relationship between the accreditor and the accredited: "Allowing JCAHO to accredit facilities that pay for surveys represent [*sic*] a conflict of interest. JCAHO's lack of objectivity plagues the current accreditation process" (Stark 1998). Stark also pointed out that, beyond this conflict of interest, JCAHO was not monitoring or upholding high enough standards for Medicare participation and had failed to identify serious problems at numerous hospitals and nursing homes (Stark 1998). The statement concludes with Stark's assertion that "the federal government has a responsibility to reevaluate the current deeming system to protect its most vulnerable citizens" (Stark 1998).

Stark's forceful remarks stemmed both from a discomfort at the lack of federal oversight of accreditation and from evidence that poor-quality hospitals and nursing homes were still being accredited. In 1999 federal investigators issued a warning that the "collegial" surveys performed by the Joint Commission were likely ineffective if the goal was to root out substandard care (Ratcliffe 2009).

The Joint Commission Today

Look around any hospital in the United States, and you will notice various signs with Joint Commission logos on them. Behind the reception desk, you may see a checklist for a staff member to consult when talking with patients and their families. The rules and policies may not have a public face, but staff are constantly presented with specific protocols and procedures that are promulgated by the Joint Commission. Because of unannounced inspections, the threat of loss of Joint Commission accreditation is ever present, and a loss of accreditation would be financially devastating for most hospitals. In short, Joint Commission standards are the law of the land for hospitals, even if they technically lack the weight of legislation. The Joint Commission now accredits more than 20,000 health care organizations. Given that there are around 6,000 hospitals currently operating in the United States, this number reflects most hospitals as well as a huge number of clinics, nursing homes, and rehabilitation centers.

The Joint Commission has a mission statement: "To continuously improve health care for the public, in collaboration with other stakeholders, by evaluating health care organizations and inspiring them to excel in providing safe and effective care of the highest quality and value" (Joint Commission 2009). The statement focuses on the commission's work of evaluation, with an additional mention of inspiration. The key stakeholder in this mission, the public, is explicit, and the process of evaluation is said to be collaborative. Although the mission emphasizes evaluation—which is, in essence, measurement—it mentions nothing about accreditation, which most health care workers and managers see as clearly the commission's role. The commission provides information to patients (known as consumers) as well as to purchasers of health care, who are most often governmental agencies and private insurance companies.

The notion of "continuous improvement," a 1999 addition to the organization's mission statement, captures a trend in health care that was borrowed from the lean production model of Toyota and other auto manufacturers; again it downplays the accrediting role of the organization, making it sound more like a consulting company than a regulator. Unsurprisingly for a mission statement, there is no hint here of the flipside of the commission's work: punitive and financially devastating consequences for any health care organization that fails to achieve commission accreditation. This focus on the positive was confirmed by an interviewee, who emphasized the role of the commission in "inspiring" hospitals.

Loss of accreditation, however, is not a likely outcome, as the commission takes its role as a consultant seriously, showing providers how to improve their organizations, and offering reinspection in certain situations. In 2002, a newspaper exposé reported that "less than 1 percent of hospitals failed to receive accreditation from the commission in the last 17 years, and some hospitals received high accreditation scores even in the midst of a public health crisis" (Berens and Japsen 2002). If loss of accreditation is an extremely unlikely outcome, then accreditation becomes potentially meaningless, something emphasized by those who have pointed out major problems in accredited hospitals.

The commission positions itself as an ally rather than an adversary of the providers it is accrediting. As a former commission president put it, "the name of the game is not to slam-dunk the institution, but to help them make changes. . . . You can't force an institution to do well. You have to provide the wherewithal to do better" (Abramowitz 1991). Indeed, the commission has dramatically increased its offerings outside the scope of, or complementary to, the accreditation process, particularly in its emphasis on clinical quality improvement and its ability to provide consulting services. The consulting services available from the Joint Commission are theoretically provided by an arm of the organization that is removed from the accreditation work, Joint Commission Resources. In practice, Joint Commission Resources can leverage vast amounts of data and experience in the services it sells to clients seeking to achieve or retain accreditation. In theory these consulting services compete with those of scores of other for profit and nonprofit consultancies, such as the Institute for Healthcare Improvement. In practice, however, it is clear that receiving advice from the same larger organization that is responsible for accreditation—and therefore your participation in the health care reimbursement system (public and private)—might be particularly desirable.

The Joint Commission is very clear about its scope and focus, and because it is the only game in town, the results of the accreditation process are used for a broad set of purposes, and the accreditation process takes on massive importance for hospitals competing for patients. As one observer of the relationship between Joint Commission measures and actual clinical quality assessed the situation, "The accreditation score and status hospitals receive from the Joint Commission on Accreditation of Healthcare Organizations' (JCAHO's) surveyors are commonly used as a surrogate assessment for quality and safety of health care. Accredited hospitals and health systems market this information, and the Centers for Medicare and Medicaid Services requires JCAHO accreditation or state accreditation for participation in Medicare. Nonetheless, it is relatively unknown to what extent JCAHO accreditation is truly associated with the quality and safety of clinical care and improved patient outcomes" (Miller et al. 2005, 240). This highlights the paradox that while commission accreditation may not be an appropriate measure of quality or patient safety, it is the only source of easily available nationally comprehensive and therefore comparable data. All the stakeholders are eager to point out the limitations of the Joint Commission's system and the commission itself is cautious in defining its scope and constraints, but no other governmental or nongovernmental agency comes close in breadth of data collection, and the Joint Commission ends up continuing its outsized role.

The commission therefore fulfills the role of a government regulator, while being technically voluntary, and operating independently. As a senior commission official told me, "independence affords us the ability to be more innovative and to talk about inspiring and evaluating, providing tools, providing guidance and moving the quality agenda, not always with a stick but with motivation and examples of, sharing stories of organizations that have succeeded and why" (personal interview 2014). Both public entities (most significantly the CMS) and private entities (all major health insurance companies) depend on the Joint Commission's stamp of approval. Centers for Medicare and Medicaid Services programs insure more than 100 million people, and therefore the CMS regulates the largest programs for purchasing health care in the country. Therefore, the dependence of the CMS on the Joint Commission accreditation confirms the mandatory nature of this requirement.

This is not an optional quality mark, like the Good Housekeeping Seal of Approval or a LEED Gold environmental rating, this is a requirement that is half-heartedly presented as a voluntary standard. According to Jost, "about two-thirds of the states base hospital licensure, in whole or in part, on Joint Commission Accreditation" (Jost 1994, 21). One commentator in the mid 1990s, before the commission was even required to reapply for its deeming power, observed that "the JCAHO is one of those obscure, private organizations that wield enormous influence in the medial community. It is the Moody's, Standard & Poor and Good Housekeeping of hospital ratings" (Schrage 1995).

According to the definition of two prominent scholars of health care and ethics, "an autonomous or self-regulating profession is one that determines which domains are primary, specifies the specific content areas and substantive criteria in each domain, and controls the procedures of accountability, especially the formal processes" (Emanuel and Emanuel 1996, 231). Some physicians are fiercely protective of this self-regulation (which is often a key aspect of professional identity). Pawlson and O'Kane write that "professionalism, along with regulation strongly influenced or controlled by professionals, has dominated accountability in medicine to a far greater degree than in virtually any other sector of our society" (2002, 200). This is unsurprising, given that doctors are the paradigmatic example of professional control of an industry (for the seminal account of the role of physicians in the creation of the US health care system, see Starr 1982). Furthermore, via the Joint Commission physicians are controlling not only the medical profession but the entire health care industry, as the commission controls much more than the credentialing of doctors. Indeed, in 1991, several cycles of attempted health care reform earlier, a retired doctor who had become a Joint Commission inspector told a group of hospital physicians that "the only response we have to the people who want to take over the medical system may be to prove that we are monitoring ourselves" (Abramowitz 1991). This attitude exemplified a notion less apparent in the commission today of its role as a protector and defender of professional power.

In more recent years, while this defensive role has still been sometimes evident, the public face of the commission emphasizes high-quality health care, patient safety, and quality improvement while minimizing the importance of doctors monitoring and regulating themselves and their workplaces. An interviewee described the commission as a "performance improvement organization," emphasizing the consulting work and the incentives from the commission standard rather than the protective role played by physician-regulators (personal interview, 2014). There are clearly inherent conflicts in physician-dominated regulation not only of their own profession but of the entire industry in which they operate.

It is worth considering what the Joint Commission's emphasis on its independence actually means. The commission prides itself on including representatives of all the major stakeholders as commissioners and on not taking orders from government. As the de facto national regulator, however, it seems that the commission could be more accurately viewed as a quasi-governmental organization because so many government agencies, specifically those that purchase or reimburse health care, explicitly depend on Joint Commission accreditation. Some agencies acquire accreditation through the process known as "deeming," which essentially means that the Joint Commission is responsible for approving organizations providing government-purchased health care. Because of this, the commission is truly independent from neither the government nor the providers it is accrediting. As one critical newspaper report angrily put it, "The nation's most influential health-care regulator frequently serves the interests of the hospital industry over those of the public, giving its seal of approval to medical centers riddled by life-threatening problems and underreporting of patient deaths due to infections and hospital errors" (Berens and Japsen 2002).

In other countries, such as the United Kingdom, evaluation and inspection of hospitals is performed by a quasi-independent commission, but the final authority for regulation lies with the government. In the United Kingdom the Care Quality Commission and its precursor organizations are ultimately accountable to the government, and they emphasize government priority areas (sometimes with a political dimension where a government has been open to attack on areas such as hospital-acquired infections or emergency room waiting times).

In the United States the government is dependent on the Joint Commission for its extensive apparatus of evaluation (which has some commonalities with the independent accrediting bodies for higher education, which designates institutions at which students are eligible for federal financial aid). The Joint Commission has a "near monopoly on hospital quality oversight" and charges hospitals tens of thousands of dollars for accreditation alone, with the possibility of additional consulting services to achieve accreditation (Moffett, Morgan, and Ashton 2005, 111). Without the Joint Commission, some other entity would need to ensure compliance with safety procedures and treatment protocols. Nevertheless, as one group of scholars put it, "the lack of public attention that JCAHO has received for their role in the quality of health care delivery is remarkable" (Moffett, Morgan, and Ashton 2005, 109).

The membership of the commission (the commissioners) demonstrates the power of health care providers. As Jost argued, "the JCAH is a private institution governed by representatives of hospitals and physicians, the participants in the health care industry who have the most to lose from competition" (Jost 1983, 839). The commission, although it has expanded its membership somewhat, continues to represent the interests of physicians and hospital groups. It is dominated by hospital administrators and physicians (many of whom are actually physician-administrators). Even the at-large nursing member is currently an administrator rather than a bedside nurse. The commission does not include a member who could reasonably be considered a patient representative. Looking at the membership of the commission it is easy to conclude that this is a cartel-like organization with an emphasis on controlling (or limiting) the supply of health care for the benefit of its providers. Theoretically, the fewer the hospitals that are accredited, the more the commission members stand to gain. Additionally, the more hospitals that seek accreditation and purchase the commission's other services, the more business the commission will also gain. Internally, the commission refers to its accredited organizations as customers, as is appropriate given that these organizations are the purchasers of its services (personal interview 2014). This terminology, however, also emphasizes that while the government, health insurers, and patients are dependent on the accrediting work of the commission, none of them are the paying customers.

Criticism of the Joint Commission

Because approval by the Joint Commission is important to health care provision, some of its main critics are not health care providers but academics, who have less to lose in voicing their critiques. Common-sense dissent is everywhere. Hospital staff constantly grumble about the foibles of the accreditors, but the published critiques tend to emanate primarily from academics who do not have a vested interest in staying on the commission's good side. A top official at the Joint Commission was very frank on this point, speaking of moving from this past, negative perception to something more positive: "This is happening more and more where we are taking that attitude [in hospitals] of fear, and the [idea that the] Joint Commission is a big bully and it just wants to ding you, to moving more toward what's consistent with our mission, which is to inspire and evaluate" (personal interview 2014).

Timothy Jost has written extensively about the apparent paradox of the government, specifically Medicare, being so heavily dependent on "private accreditation" (Jost 1983, 1994). He states that "given the importance of assuring quality of Medicare-financed institutional health care, it is remarkable that throughout its existence Medicare has depended on a private organization to fulfill this [quality assurance] function" (1994, 22). Indeed, the Joint Commission's more recent work overseas notwithstanding, other countries do not leave this essential task to nongovernmental organizations. Jost rightly points out that the government is delegating the regulation of health care providers to an organization founded and controlled by the providers themselves, allowing for what amounts to self-regulation.

The commission is not open to public (political or patient) scrutiny or influence. As Jost writes, "JCAH lacks the saving grace of availability for achieving public policy goals other than efficiency. It is not open to public scrutiny, participation or responsibility" (1983, 883). This is in stark contrast to the quality regulator in the United Kingdom (known as the Care Quality Commission at the time of writing), which is sometimes accused of being open to too much political influence, with standards sometimes reflecting specific hot-button political issues such as waiting times for appointments with specialists and ever-changing targets ultimately determined by the government.

It is worth noting that even those relatively well-versed in the US health care economy may have trouble distinguishing between the work of the Joint Commission and the CMS, and between public and private regulators. Given that many supposedly voluntary standards have become required for meaningful participation in the selling of health care, the distinctions between mandatory and voluntary standards become somewhat obtuse. As Moffett and colleagues put it, "JCAHO has received much criticism for the accreditation process. Much of the commentary, while directed at JCAHO, is actually a reflection of the CMS-JCAHO relationship" (2005, 113). In an interview, I asked a Joint Commission official about this relationship, and the response was quite illuminating:

> Government relationships are very interesting. Medicare or CMS is the governmental agency that authorizes the Joint Commission every 6 years, through an application process, to have deeming authority over our organizations that we accredit, meaning if you are accredited for deeming purposes at the Joint Commission you are then certified to receive payment from Medicaid and Medicare services. The majority of our hospital organizations use Joint Commission accreditation for deeming so it does [provide] an additional value but also pressure to the organization to do well on the survey. We are overseen by CMS, they do a valid validation survey to calculate and estimate how well we have done after we have evaluated an organization. They audit our records, they evaluate how we evaluate complaints and our surveys. So there's a whole process of oversight that CMS has over the Joint Commission. (Personal interview 2014)

This oversight, however, is buried deep in the black box of the Joint Commission, and the widespread perception is that the commission sets the regulatory standards and that the CMS accept these standards (personal interviews 2012–14).

The domination of the Joint Commission by physicians is a problem because other stakeholders may be underrepresented and doctors themselves face a complex set of interests and incentives. As early as the late 1990s, scholars were concerned about the double-agent role that doctors assume by attempting to serve multiple stakeholders. They argued that accountability procedures "must motivate appropriate physician behavior in a way that acknowledges professional principles and peer respect, while at the same time meeting the needs of patients, purchasers, and other external groups" (Shortell 1998, 1107). The relatively minor changes in the role of the Joint Commission, specifically in its relationship with the CMS, which I will discuss, have done little to change the incentives or to modify the decisive role of physicians in the commission.

Implementing Change through the Joint Commission

In an article examining the relationship between the implementation of Joint Commission quality improvement programs and actual improvement of clinical outcomes, Weiner et al. (2006) focus on the process of implementation. They define implementation as "the transition period, following a decision to adopt a new idea or practice, when intended users put that new idea or practice into use" (Weiner et al. 2006, 308). It is notable that this decision may not be made by the hospital staff or management but by the commission. Confirming my central assertion in this book, Weiner and colleagues found that staff involvement was a major and significant determination of the successful implementation of change in hospitals, in this case for quality improvement programs leading to improved clinical outcomes. Crucially, these authors found that depth (staff involvement) led to successful programs while breadth (attempted implementation across multiple units within a hospital) was associated with failed implementation.

Information from Joint Commission leaders suggests that staff involvement is not central to the creation or implementation of their standards. Rather, these standards come from above and de-emphasize input from frontline providers. Instead, the standards are evidence-based but are created by commissioners and the research arm of the commission. Although a standard may be modified after field-testing, a high-level Joint Commission officer informed me that she could not think of a single example where a new or modified standard had been initiated in a hospital workplace. In fact, this interviewee was concerned that frontline workers and hospitals overemphasize quick fixes rather than more difficult evidence-based solutions, such as those promulgated by the Joint Commission: "Hospitals love . . . checklists and bundles and those kind of things spread like wildfire. There tends to be a desire among hospitals to get a quick fix on a problem, and one of the things that the Joint Commission does is think about how difficult it is to adopt a solution for a complex problem from one organization to another because no two organizations are alike" (personal interview 2014).

Instead, this official emphasized the scope (although quite limited) for input once a standard has been created at the top: "When we are developing new standards we field test and field review those surveys so that our customer could comment and advise as to the practicality and identify the potential burdens, unnecessary burdens that the requirements can impose on an organization. And that feedback is really used to decide whether to move forward or whether to modify a standard" (personal interview 2014). This interviewee also spoke about outreach from the commission to its customers as focused on executives and physician leaders.

It is also clear that the Joint Commission believes itself to sometimes be the bitter medicine that a hospital must take in order to improve patient care and safety. As an interviewee said:

> In a highly complex industry you need to reduce variation as much as possible, and that's what the Joint Commission standards do, they reduce variation. And if you believe in some of the principles of what drives risk, variation drives risk, so reducing variation and thereby reducing some risk does bring some benefits to the organization even though they may be appearing as cumbersome initially. Everything that's introduced to an organization is always, because of the change challenge and change management, if you like, is always burdensome. It's only after these changes have been fully adopted and have been integrated into the workplace do they become manageable and no longer burdensome. (Personal interview 2014)

The Joint Commission's authority is a form of industry self-regulation with the attendant strengths and weaknesses (Gunningham and Rees 1997), but it has been given the status of quasi-government regulator. This allows the commission to emphasize its independence when useful but to operate with the clout of a government regulator in the majority of its work. It is clear from my interviews and voluminous other material that hospitals treat the commission as a government regulator—one that ultimately determines the fate of any hospital (Jost 1983).

Government Regulation through Purchasing: The Case of the Centers for Medicare and Medicaid Services

The CMS is the federal agency charged with administering Medicare and Medicaid—that is, for spending the program-budgeted money on actual health care for the relevant populations. Through its role in administering Medicare and Medicaid as well as the State Children's Health Insurance Plan (known as CHIP or S-CHIP), the agency purchases more than $500 billion in health care each year on behalf of a staggering number of people—100 million (Centers for Medicare and Medicaid Services Office of Public Affairs 2012). The CMS works as both the regulator and the purchaser for these federally funded health care programs, although some of the regulatory work is essentially outsourced to the Joint Commission. As Moffett and colleagues put it, "JCAHO's near monopoly is a result [of] its relations with CMS directly through Medicare and indirectly through residency requirements" (2005, 111).[2] Astonishingly, although it exists in a country without single-payer health care, the CMS is the largest purchaser of health care in the world (Iglehart 2001). It becomes clear, then, how this massive health care purchaser's choice of regulating or accrediting agency might have an enormous impact on the health care industry as a whole, including care purchased by non-CMS entities such as private health insurers.

As early as 1977, when the agency was relatively young, it was clear that the clout the CMS held as a purchaser effectively meant there was public control over privately run hospitals (Weiner 1977). Because the CMS dictated the acceptable costs of various health care services and because no provider

---

2. Joint Commission accreditation is essentially required for hospitals to participate in Graduate Medical Education programs (i.e., medical residencies), as determined by the Accreditation Council for Graduate Medical Education (ACGME). While recent revisions to ACGME make it technically possible to host medical residents without Joint Commission accreditation, in practice there is little incentive or advantage for hospitals to pursue another, more complex route (Accreditation Council for Graduate Medical Education 2010, 4).

could afford to operate without serving this huge segment of the population, the CMS began to set the price for health care. More than a decade ago, after the failed Clinton attempt at health care reform and before the more successful Obama reform, John Iglehart, the founder of *Health Affairs* magazine, wrote,

> There have always been conflicts between the CMS and its predecessors, on the one hand, and physicians, hospitals, clinical laboratories, home health agencies, kidney dialysis centers, and suppliers of durable medical equipment, on the other. Medicare is the largest single source of income for all these groups. No amount of regulatory relief will entirely erase these inherent conflicts. The CMS has a fiduciary role as guardian of tax revenues that represent 15 percent of the federal budget. Legislators, the medical profession, and health care organizations have questioned the agency's ability to manage its vast domain. (Iglehart 2001)

The evidence from my interviews shows that there is a spillover effect from CMS regulation. Technically, hospitals could follow different protocols and procedures for patients whose care is funded through CMS programs than those provided for privately insured patients. But in reality this does not happen. In practice, hospitals create systems to comply with the rules and regulations of the CMS and use these systems for all patients. It would not make sense to have two separate sets of paperwork and procedures. Thus, as with the Joint Commission, there is a set of regulations that is applied nationally. When the CMS mandates that hospitals change their procedures, hospitals must make the required changes or jeopardize a large portion of their budgets.

Perhaps the most profound way that the CMS promulgates change on the front line is through the reimbursement system. Reimbursement for Medicaid and Medicare services is deeply complex and sets the framework of financial incentives for hospitals. There has been a great deal of criticism of the programs for incentivizing the quantity but not the quality of care. In particular, the role of Medicare reimbursement in driving decisions by health care providers has come under a great deal of criticism (Berwick et al. 2003). Many commentators have noted that reimbursement was driving health care while the reverse would be more desirable, but this problem proved intractable for many years. The ways in which Medicare (as federally specified) drove the provision of care show that health care was truly federally controlled and that bottom-up change was impossible without top-down changes to the payment system.

Even a relatively modest change to the reimbursement system can cause changes in decisions on the front line. Again and again, it has become clear that hospitals and their staffs are unable to make decisions based only on prioritizing high-quality care. Cost is always a factor, sometimes at the expense of quality. In 1997 Congress passed the Balanced Budget Act, after an election battle that focused on reducing the deficit at all costs. The act cut numerous areas of government spending, one of which was Medicare. The cut to Medicare was a reduction in payment for numerous specific procedures as well as cuts to annual increases (equivalent to cost-of-living increases) for certain work (for a more detailed account of some of the specific payment reductions, see Lindrooth et al. 2006). Taken together, these reductions cut the budgets of many hospitals significantly, especially hospitals that received a high number of Medicare payments, which tend disproportionately to be public or so-called safety net hospitals. Indeed, the cuts proved to be so drastic that much of the funding had to be restored by Congress in 1999 (Lindrooth et al. 2006).

After such a dramatic change in reimbursement, scholars were able to trace the effect of budget reduction on the level of nurse staffing in hospitals that earned the highest proportion of their income from Medicare payments (Lindrooth et al. 2006). Their analysis demonstrated that the lower reimbursement rate led to higher nurse–patient ratios: fewer nurses per patient. Some authors found it difficult to use these particular data to draw specific connections with quality of care; however, others, looking more specifically at the relationship between nurse–patient ratios and care quality, found that the higher ratios had a direct, negative impact on the quality of patient care (Aiken, Clarke, and Sloane 2002; Aiken et al. 2002; Gordon, Buchanan, and Bretherton 2008). It is clear then, that a change in reimbursement, in this case to serve the purely political objective of balancing the federal budget, affected the provision of care in hospitals and had the potential to change both the processes and outcomes of patient care.

The decisive role of reimbursement rates and rules has been noted for some time. Indeed, this problem in the US health care system is an issue in the quality of care for those whose care is funded by government programs and by private, for-profit insurance companies (Brownlee 2008). In an open letter published in *Health Affairs* in 2003, fifteen advocates—renowned physicians, economists, and other experienced professionals, including Donald Berwick and Nancy-Ann Deparle, who became key players in the Obama administration's health care team—called for immediate reform of the Medicare reimbursement system, with an emphasis on payments based on outcomes. These commentators forcefully argued that the unacceptable number of medical errors and the deep flaws in the quality of care could not be improved without deep changes to the reimbursement systems:

> Despite a few initial successes, the inertia of the health system could easily overwhelm nascent efforts to raise average performance levels out of mediocrity. At issue is not the dedication of health professionals but the lack of systems—including information systems—that reduce error and reinforce best practices, as such systems do in other industries such as aviation and nuclear power. We have concluded that such systematic changes will not come forth quickly enough unless strong financial incentives are offered to get the attention of managers and governing boards. As the biggest purchaser in the system, the Medicare program should take the lead in this regard. Decisive change will occur only when Medicare, with the full support of the administration and Congress, creates financial incentives that promote pursuit of improved quality. (Berwick et al. 2003)

The influential members of this group believe that reimbursement systems drive health care decisions, not the other way around. It took many years, until the passage of the Affordable Care Act of 2010 under Obama, for meaningful movement in this direction, and the complexity of the reimbursement rules and regulations means that changes will be slow and ultimately subject to ongoing wrangling over implementation driven by stakeholders with potentially divergent interests.

It is noteworthy that changes in reimbursement are the main mechanism the federal government has for delivery system reform, whether to cut costs, improve care quality, or both (Rosenthal 2007). Because the federal government has not shown an ability to significantly influence the Joint Commission's accreditation process but instead chooses to accept the accreditation rules as given, it could theoretically work outside of accreditation to create or incentivize change. But the key area of reimbursement is also outsourced to powerful private organizations controlled by physicians (primarily the American Medical Association through its ownership of the coding system used in medical billing). Although hospitals are nominally autonomous and able to deliver care in any manner they choose, the reimbursement rules combined with the de facto mandatory accreditation process make specific practices and procedures the only viable options, and this creates uniform national regulation not unlike the British system. The primary contrast with the UK regulatory regime is that the US system is driven by payment systems that create a set of detailed financial rules and incentives, rather than the absolute rules in the United Kingdom that are focused on best practice rather than reimbursement.

Combined Effect of De Facto Regulation Systems

The CMS allows the Joint Commission to retain its near monopoly on accreditation through the use of deemed status. Rather than being accredited by the CMS itself, an organization is deemed to be acceptable because of its accreditation by a voluntary regulator, which is almost always the Joint Commission. This theoretically optional subcontracting of accreditation keeps the CMS control at arm's length. The Joint Commission is so entwined with accrediting Medicare and Medicaid providers that it was initially granted its accrediting authority in the 1965 law without going through any review process (other putative accreditors have always been required to go through an approval process with the CMS before being granted deeming authority).

At the time Medicare and Medicaid were established, JCAH (the Joint Commission's acronym at that time) was the only expert body on health care quality or accreditation standards, so making commission accreditation the simplest route to the so-called conditions of participation in the new government health care programs seemed efficient and logical: "[The 1965] Act granted the Joint Commission a unique status to deem hospitals as eligible for Medicare payments with little federal oversight. Through the Social Security Act of 1965, Congress, on its own cognizance, granted this deemed status that limited the executive branch's authority over the accreditation process. The Joint Commission had not sought it out; nor was it aware of this statutory provision when it was being framed" (Menendez 2010, 71). Although the Social Security Act did require some ongoing validation of accreditation, the consensus is that the commission was able to operate autonomously for more than four decades (Menendez 2010).

The special status of the Joint Commission remained in place from 1965 until 2008, when the Medicare Improvements for Patients and Providers Act required that the commission be treated like other accreditors, and the commission therefore had to apply for renewal of deeming status (Joint Commission 2008). In its official statement on the new law, the commission stated, somewhat equivocally, that "in principle, The Joint Commission generally supports the provision's intention" (Joint Commission 2008). Because there was little rationale for the Joint Commission's privileged position in accrediting, the commission could hardly argue with the new law; in practice, it has continued to dominate the accreditation of hospitals even with the new supposedly level playing field among aspiring accreditors.

To untangle the relationship between the CMS and the Joint Commission, it is necessary to understand why and how the commission lost its privileged status as essentially the deemer of record. As one hospital administrator puts it, "[the] legislation was reportedly justified by a critical concern about the Joint Commission's ability to ensure patient safety through its hospital accreditation program. In actuality, the change in the Medicare law was spearheaded by an assertive congressman advocating for increased CMS authority over the Joint Commission" (Menendez 2010, 70). Juliet Menendez, a nurse and hospital administrator with responsibility for quality, argued against the legislated change on two grounds: first, that it was politically motivated and poorly justified, and second, that it created an undue burden on hospitals that had to comply with revamped Joint Commission standards (Menendez 2010).

In 2004, as the patient-safety movement was gaining influence, members of Congress requested a Government Accountability Office (GAO) report on patient safety (and the oversight thereof) in hospitals. The GAO report clearly recommended that the Joint Commission should not have its privileged status but should be required to apply for its deeming authority like all other accreditors across the health care sector (US Government Accountability Office 2004). This report contained numerous criticisms of the Joint Commission, particularly regarding discrepancies between commission reports and state agency surveys. Until this time, Joint Commission visits to hospitals were announced ahead of time, which for obvious reasons is no longer the case. The commission now makes unannounced surveys eighteen to thirty-nine months after its initial survey in each accreditation cycle (Joint

Commission 2011). The inconsistencies between Joint Commission reports and the results of state surveys led the GAO report to conclude that the commission should not continue its special status. In comments on a draft that were incorporated into the final report, JCAHO (as its acronym was then) and others criticized the methodology of the report and argued that the flaws in the commission's accreditation process were overblown and misrepresented (Menendez 2010; US Government Accountability Office 2004). Ultimately, however, "JCAHO stated that it did not object to [GAO's] matter for congressional consideration that CMS be given the same oversight authority over JCAHO's hospital accreditation program that it has over other health care accreditation programs" (US Government Accountability Office 2004). The nonexistent rationale for this longstanding special status, combined with the commission's confidence that it could retain its deeming authority even under the new rules, made its acquiescence to the new law the only logical and politically safe course of action.

Chapter 5

PUSHING BACK FROM THE FRONT LINE

Staff Responses to Privatization in the National Health Service

When change is imposed on a hospital from above, frontline staff sometimes push back. Workers and their unions may be unable to halt a major policy change, but they may be able to fight back as the new policy takes effect. A policy may be passed by a legislative body, but the actual implementation is still subject to the interests and influence of the workplace stakeholders. This was the case in the United Kingdom when a new form of hospital financing and operation was introduced, initially by the Conservative government of the early 1990s (Broadbent and Laughlin 2005). Unions representing frontline staff fought off the most damaging aspects of the new initiative, ultimately forcing a change in national policy. This became a demonstration of a policy feedback loop: frontline workers, after experiencing the change in policy, pushed for changes, which were eventually implemented nationwide. In this case, the policy was that of neoliberalism, privatization, and increased competition—a force that has become a permanent fixture in both the United Kingdom and the United States. The backlash or resistance, however, was critical, and as the neoliberal policies became more widespread, the pushback from frontline workers became more organized and more effective.[1]

Since the mid-1980s, public services in the United Kingdom have undergone a process of marketization. This has included various forms of internal competition and outsourcing as well as wholesale privatization (for example, of the public utilities). The most widespread form of marketization has been the Private Finance Initiative (PFI), introduced in the mid-1990s. This program created a hybrid form of financing for public-private facilities and adopted this financing for hospitals, schools, and prisons. The initiative was enacted through legislation during the Conservative governments of the 1990s, but its use accelerated rapidly when Tony Blair's New Labour government came to power in 1997. Under the PFI, facilities such as hospitals but also schools and prisons are built by private contractors with private money providing the up-front financing for a long-term loan to the government. The facilities are then operated in partnership with the public sector. When this arrangement is used to procure public services, a private sector consortium is contracted to finance, build, and operate a hospital or community services, and the client makes an agreed annual payment for the duration of the contract (typically thirty years, but sometimes much longer). The consortium creates a series of contractual and equity arrangements between a financial institution to secure financing, a construction company to build the facility, and a facilities management company to maintain the building and provide support services over the lifetime of the contract. When a PFI is applied to a hospital in the United Kingdom, the National Health Service (NHS) hospital makes an agreed annual payment for the duration of the contract, and this represents the first obligation on a trust's revenue.

The PFI is now the primary method of procuring major public sector assets such as hospitals in the United Kingdom, although the Labour governments under prime ministers Blair and Brown generally preferred to use the more neutral sounding term "public-private partnerships." As of 2009, the Department of Health had built one hundred and one hospital and commu-

---

1. This chapter is based on three years of intensive research (with more targeted follow-up interviews after the initial work), by Stephen Bach and myself, including in-depth case studies in hospitals and interviews with key stakeholders at the national and regional levels. The research was conducted jointly, and specific findings from it have been published elsewhere (Bach and Givan, 2005, 2010; Givan and Bach 2007).

nity health facilities using the PFI (HM Treasury 2009); since 1997, only a handful of hospitals have been built through conventional public financing. The imposition of this form of financing and operation of new hospitals, once in place, was not something that workers or their unions could stop, and the operation of these hospitals was constantly subject to new pressures and constraints. Despite its high public profile, there was initially little political interest in the workforce consequences of the PFI, with many parliamentary inquiries neglecting workforce issues (UNISON 2009a). Instead, politicians focused on whether these initiatives could provide increased health service capacity at a reasonable cost.

To illustrate the feedback effects stemming directly from a policy change, in this chapter I draw on core data from a multiyear case study of the workforce consequences of the PFI, conducted jointly with Stephen Bach. The hospital in this case, for which I use the pseudonym Greenbelt, was viewed as a flagship hospital project by policymakers, investors, and some union representatives. Unlike some PFI hospitals that had serious operational problems from their inception, this hospital was widely perceived to be a success story, representing a smooth transition to public-private hospital financing. One of the first PFI projects completed after the Labour government took power in 1997, it gained a high public profile, and it was a frequent reference point in ongoing discussions of the value of the PFI. In this case, the new form of hospital financing and operation led to pushback from frontline staff and unions, which in turn led to a further policy change. The change resulting from this feedback improved working conditions for privatized staff and eliminated on a nationwide basis the so-called two-tier workforce in which employees doing the same work in the same workplace received unequal pay and conditions.

Policies and Politics

In a PFI contract, a wide range of support services are outsourced, and these services are frequently bundled into a single facilities management agreement. These services tend to include such services as food service, cleaning, parking, maintenance, and laundry. These agreements detail a guaranteed level of service from the private company and a guaranteed payment from the government to the private contractor. For example, the contract might specify benchmarks for the quality, quantity and cleanliness of hospital linens.

Despite originally labeling the PFI a form of privatization (something to which it had once been staunchly opposed), the Labour government, elected in 1997, was a staunch advocate of bringing in specialist private sector expertise. Encouraging partnerships was attractive to this government, which was attempting to distance itself from the low-trust models of outsourcing favored by previous Conservative governments (Grimshaw, Vincent, and Willmott 2002). The Confederation of British Industry, an equivalent to the US Chamber of Commerce, also has argued that public-private partnerships can offer win-win outcomes in which private employers can profit from the contracts with no detriment to the workers (Confederation of British Industry 2006).

Prime Minister Tony Blair consistently argued that he was not ideologically wedded to either public or private sector provision of public services. Instead, he claimed that "what matters is what works." Blair argued that the determining factor would be the quality and efficiency of the services rather than who was providing them. Although many union activists privately, and sometimes publicly, stated that they believed Blair was in fact strongly in favor of privatization, Blair himself always claimed that his position was purely pragmatic.

At a time when subcontracting to the private sector was already widespread in the public services, the real novelty of the PFI was its mode of financing, combined with the long-term contracts given to private companies. Private sector financing allowed the provision of public services without large up-front costs on the public balance sheet. Tony Blair argued that "we cannot make sustained investment in funding for schools, hospitals and rail without fiscal discipline" (Blair 2002, 13). Blair presented the PFI as the only way to build new schools and hospitals.

Trade Union Responses to Marketization

Many of the unions' concerns about staff reductions, which had been voiced under previous forms of outsourcing, re-emerged with the advent of the PFI. Several large general unions were strongly opposed to the PFI, but it was hard for them to mobilize widespread opposition for three reasons. First, the program was supported by both major political parties, which gave the unions little political leverage on the issue. Second, the PFI process was highly technical, involving specialized financing and accounting practices; it was more difficult to mobilize support against complex, often opaque, policies. Finally, the PFI funding process allowed the government to build much needed new facilities such as schools and hospitals. Communities where the schools and hospitals were old and poorly maintained were desperate to have new buildings, so they were not overly concerned about the specifics of the financial arrangements.

Union opposition to PFI schemes was initially both ideological and pragmatic. Many unions argued that, as a matter of a principle, public services paid for with tax money should not generate profits for private companies. The unions were also concerned that privatized employees would be paid less and receive less favorable conditions and benefits. The unions that opposed the PFI most vociferously were those whose members (or potential future members) were likely to face privatization. The unions representing only doctors or nurses took a much less public stance on the issue because PFI hospitals did not directly affect their members, or at least did not introduce new private sector employers. The unions representing only the clinical staff such as nurses first saw the new hospitals as merely new facilities, often replacing crumbling, century-old hospitals. It took some time for them to understand that even though their staff and their work were not being transferred to private employers, the effects of these contracts on all staff were profound. The PFI would illustrate a specific case of employee constraints on the implementation of change in the workplace.

In the NHS, the trade union responses to the PFI demonstrated the continuity and resilience of individual union strategies, even in a rapidly changing political and workplace context. In the case of the PFI, the Labour government was unable to command the support of the unions at the policymaking level and only sporadically achieved employee support at the point of implementation in the workplace. As such, PFI implementation was piecemeal and widely varied. Union employees in the workplace were able to shape the ways in which reform policies were implemented, even if their representative organizations were relatively powerless to affect the policy itself. This impact on implementation could then feed back into revisions of the policy.

Union responses to the PFI fell into two main categories. The more general unions (such as UNISON and the GMB, two of the largest public services unions) fought well-resourced campaigns against the PFI as a matter of principle. The GMB and UNISON both represented many members whose work was transferred to private companies, who were thus directly affected by these schemes. These two unions mounted broad campaigns against the PFI in the political and public arena. UNISON argued that the PFI was antithetical to the public service ethos. Their argument was that publicly financed and provided services were inherently of a higher quality than private services because of the dedication and altruism of those who provide them, and that a profit motive creates different priorities and incentives that result in inferior service quality. UNISON claimed that private sector employees providing public services might "find that there are conflicts between fulfilling their public service obligations and their corporate obligations" (UNISON 2002b, 11). This public service ethos was sometimes linked to a professional ethic among doctors and nurses (Dixon, Le Grand, and Smith 2003, 4). For unions, the fear was that PFI companies would prioritize "profit before care" (Royal College of Nursing 2000). Indeed, with the increasingly widespread private provision of public services, the House of Commons Public Administration Select Committee launched an investigation into the public service ethos (Public Administration Select Committee 2002). One complication in the unions' position, however, was that it is difficult for unions to promote the notion of a public sector ethos without also implying that these dedicated staff are willing to work for inferior pay and conditions (personal interview 2002).

The other large general union, the GMB, also developed a broad anti-PFI campaign under the title Keep Public Service Public. This campaign featured general outreach in the form of newspaper advertising that emphasized the poor employment practices and high levels of executive compensation of the major PFI contractors (GMB 2002b). One GMB official highlighted the union's disappointment that Labour had so enthusiastically embraced the PFI, stating that "we had been given assurances by government when in opposition that [it] would change, it hasn't, it's got worse" (personal interview 2002). This union official also freely admitted that there was a competitive edge to the campaign: both UNISON and the GMB wished to appear as the most effective and active anti-PFI union.

At the local level, however, the response was more mixed as the unions, realizing that they were unlikely to change national policy, were forced to respond to the PFIs and work with the private companies who were now employing their members. As one national officer stated, "We have a twin track approach, which means we can challenge policies fundamentally [and] at the same time do whatever we need to do to protect our members" (personal interview 2004). The unions needed to focus on the point of implementation, especially when union influence on policy and legislation was minimal.

The second type of union response was more muted and deliberate. The professional unions such as those representing nurses and teachers took a much less proactive approach to the PFIs because core professional employment, such as that of teachers, physicians, and nurses, was not being transferred to the private sector. Although the new facilities provided their working environment, the terms and conditions of employment for these professional union members remained unchanged, so the effect on them was less direct. Their unions were both slower and more pragmatic in formulating responses to the PFI, both as a national policy and in practice.

Thus, the general unions fought the PFI both at the political level and in the workplace, while the professional unions addressed the initiative only once it reached the stage of implementation. The PFI was both a symptom and a cause of friction in the relationship between the unions and the governing Labour party. It obviously caused friction, but the willingness of the Labour government to continue the program against the vociferous objection of public sector unions demonstrated how little the government relied on the unions for support, a big change from the earlier days of the Labour Party. The PFI brought out the major differences in types of unions in the UK public sector, specifically in the NHS, and their varying abilities to enable or constrain workplace change. The differences in the responses from the professional, nonpolitical unions and the general, politically affiliated unions were even more pronounced in addressing the PFI as a policy issue than as a workplace issue.

Unions that fought PFI in principle on the national level generally did so based on two arguments: first, the PFI was unacceptable because it allowed private companies to profit from public services; second, in practice the PFI did not work and was not fair to the affected employees. The second argument depended on evidence from actual experience with the PFI, but the case for the first argument could be made in the abstract as it relied on a principle rather than a pragmatic evaluation of the program. This rhetoric was a bold rejection of "What matters is what works," Tony Blair's mantra for public service reform (Wintour 2002).

Some trade unions critical of PFI schemes raised concerns about poor working conditions, inadequate training, and declining service standards (British Medical Association 2009; UNISON 2005a, 2005b). Despite these strong criticisms, trade unions had trouble orchestrating opposition because of the complexity of the PFI contracts and their appeal to the workforce (Ruane 2000). When the PFI was presented as the only way for a crumbling hospital to be replaced, it was difficult for unions to rally local opposition to the new building. This was especially the case when the hospitals to be replaced were more than a century old and often featured long, large wards that housed thirty or more patients with little privacy. The allure of a new, modern facility to hospital staff and the local community was undeniable.

The unions that most actively campaigned against the PFI were those whose employees were most directly affected. Two of the largest public service unions, UNISON and the GMB, mounted high-profile national campaigns against the PFI specifically, and the private provision of public services more generally. UNISON's Positively Public campaign and the GMB's Keep Public Services Public campaign both worked toward similar goals of public provision and financing of public services. These public campaigns were backed by negotiations between public service unions and the Labour government over the specifics of employment transfers and the rights of employees affected by PFI schemes.

Workplace Consequences

In the workplace, privatization had real, everyday consequences because if facilities or support services were inadequate, patient care would suffer. The consequences of the PFI prompted a good deal of give and take in the workplace. As one PFI investor stated, "One of the best things that PFI has done is that it has broken down some of the barriers between the two sectors. Private sector [companies] think public sector is all flabby; public sector think we [are] all Rachman [a notoriously evil slum lord] type figures. PFI is forcing the two sectors to speak to each other more. . . . People [are] starting to understand that neither side is quite as different as people thought, or quite as bad" (personal interview 2003).

The unions had to make adjustments. Although several unions consistently opposed the PFI as a policy, at the local level they had to work within the constraints of the PFIs that had already been implemented. As Mick Carpenter put it, the PFI "is opposed in principle [by UNISON] and calls are made to retain public ownership and find alternative means of funding capital projects. At the same time, in practice considerable effort has been made at the national and local levels to influence the terms of the PFI" (Carpenter 2000, 207). One GMB official stated succinctly, "We follow the work" (personal interview 2004). The general unions could not afford to ignore the staff who were transferred out of the public sector, or they risked a significant loss of membership (as many unions suffered during the era of mass privatization and outsourcing in the 1980s). The initiative required a great deal of attention from unions as they faced the transfer of staff to a new employer and new (sometimes inadequate) facilities for thousands of employees. The general unions responded rapidly to implementation issues (led by their national campaigns and available resources), while the professional unions frequently had to play catch-up because they were less prepared for the workplace problems that consistently emerged.

Union responses to the PFI in the workplace consisted of addressing issues as they occurred and facilitating communication between NHS staff, private facilities management companies, and NHS hospital trust management. Workplace responses to the PFI were both practical and reactive, focusing on narrow, specific problems rather than the broader ideological or political concerns. Unions had to address a range of employee concerns from those already working in PFI hospitals and from those at earlier stages in the PFI process. These ranged from minor problems such as issues with special meals from caterers (one interviewee spoke of a hospital caterer who could not offer kosher meals) to major design problems such as wards too narrow to accommodate the necessary beds and equipment (personal interview 2004).

Local union officers often took on key roles as disseminators of information, plugging the accountability and information gaps in the PFI hospitals. The experience with the PFI suggested that there were few successful channels of accountability for the private contractors. Often union officers would take on the role of intermediaries, reporting facilities problems to the trust management when the private contractor failed to resolve a problem. Union representatives, up to the level of regional officers, frequently served as the key links in solving operational problems and bridging communication gaps between frontline staff, private managers, and hospital administrators.

Similarly, when staff members were frustrated by a lack of responsiveness from trust management and facilities management, they often brought their concerns and complaints to their union officers (various personal interviews, 2003–5). As one union representative stated, after complaints had been brought to the private management company, "nothing ever gets done" (personal interview 2004). Nevertheless, efforts were being made to smooth the implementation of the reform program. The employees could not stop the private financing of a hospital once it was under contract, but they could try to ensure that the hospital functioned as well as possible and provided high-quality health care (Public Administration Select Committee 2002).

In PFI hospitals, much of the day-to-day union work consisted of troubleshooting, highlighting problems such as inadequate cleaning and catering or disregard for infection control procedures. Health and safety concerns, for both patients and staff, were often brought to light by union representatives when hospital managers were unaware of problems. Union stewards worked as troubleshooters, constantly bringing problems to the attention of the responsible parties and attempting to resolve issues that fell through the gap between the public managers and the PFI consortium, such as lack of communication between hospital managers and contractor employees regarding custodial work and working conditions. Although problems with poor design were widespread and heavily publicized in the early PFI hospitals (especially in the Cumberland Infirmary, the first PFI hospital to open), once the hospitals had been built, the unions focused on the problems that could feasibly be corrected (for much more on the problems at the Cumberland Infirmary, see Commission for Health Improvement 2003a; Lister 2003).

The unions played a critical role in allowing the hospitals to function and in overcoming initial operational problems such as how and when to use the hotline through which hospital staff were supposed to report any problems with the operation of the building. Without the voice of union members and representatives, the PFI hospitals would have been susceptible to all kinds of problems, from cross-infection to diminished bed capacity. The interviewees I spoke with believed that the hospitals would not have been able to function without the extra effort exerted by the unions and their members in providing high-quality care and troubleshooting.

Traditionally, in NHS hospitals the ward staff worked as a team, usually under the supervision of a matron, a senior nurse-manager. The team included both professional and support staff. Teams were kept together and assigned to a specific ward, and the staff had a high degree of coordination and information sharing. My interviewees spoke of the collegiality and sense of common purpose that arose from these ward teams. The disintegration of any semblance of a ward team in the PFI hospitals was a key concern to nursing staff (although staff across the NHS stated that the rise of outsourcing in the 1980s had severely damaged ward teams as well). With the ancillary service workers employed by a private company (or sometimes by one or more temporary agencies under contract to the private employer), the nursing staff felt unable to build relationships with these workers and ensure high service quality. One nurse, for example, stated that an "issue for us is that the support staff are no longer NHS employees. They have such a huge turnover of staff that these people don't have a chance to become members of the ward team" (Lister 2003, 23). Many nurses raised concerns about the high turnover of cleaning staff and the consequences of this problem for hygiene and infection. My interviewees believed that this detachment of ancillary staff led to inferior patient care. The Royal College of Nursing (RCN), in particular, wanted to address this as an area of professional concern. It did not, however, campaign nationally or locally, and the situation remains relatively unchanged today. My interviewees specifically mentioned that when the uniforms for subcontracted staff are recognizably different, it undermines any feeling of belonging to a single team.

In the workplace, the responses to the PFI were similar among both professional and general unions. Concerns from the workplace filtered up to national conferences through resolutions proposed by the local branches and their frontline members. The key difference among the unions, however, was the level of resources and support available from the union headquarters, and successful local action for unions was dependent on resources from the unions' national and regional offices. For example, UNISON and the GMB provided support, advice, and research since the inception of the PFI; UNISON developed a one-day course specifically for members campaigning against PFI locally. The RCN only began providing detailed information to members and local representatives much later, and they took much longer to offer training and information days to the affected members.

The role of union officers in disseminating and conveying information regarding problems in the functioning of the hospitals largely determined whether unions could make changes in the workplace. By identifying problems, officers and lay representatives (who were usually frontline staff) had more influence on and insight into the most appropriate solutions to the problems. Although staff concerns, even when taken up by unions, were not always addressed by management, this key role of union officers did constrain the implementation of the PFI, by identifying which employees could improve the day-to-day functioning of the hospital.

It proved difficult for trade unions to prevent marketization and the use of the PFI in the NHS (Ruane 2000). This led the unions to adopt a "a more pragmatic, twin-track approach in the face of a growth in private sector involvement and relatively low union membership density, and significant recruitment potential in parts of the private sector" (Wing 2003, 3). The unions supplemented their ideological opposition to the PFI with a more pragmatic strategy that focused on organizing the private sector (subcontracted) workers and securing decent pay and conditions for them that were similar to those in the public sector.

Crucially, after the implementation of many large PFI schemes, trade unions campaigned successfully to ensure some re-regulation of employment conditions to end the creation of a two-tier workforce. Although NHS staff who were transferred to the private sector were covered by the Transfer of Undertakings (Protection of Employment) Regulations 1981 (TUPE), this provided only limited protection. TUPE excluded pension rights and provided no defense against subsequent changes for new staff (Davies 2004). Much as unions in the United States have been forced to "sell out their unborn" and accept poorer pay and benefits for new employees, existing union members in the United Kingdom had to decide whether to take a stand to defend the new, private sector employees who were providing support services for public agencies.

In 2005, the unions, employers, and the Department of Health reached an agreement with private contractors that up to 30,000 hospital cleaners, porters, and catering staff working for private contractors in the NHS would receive pay and conditions "no less favorable" than the national pay agreement between the trade unions and the Department of Health. The costs of implementation were divided between NHS hospitals who were provided with some additional resources and the relevant private contractors (Department of Health 2007). The NHS trusts and private contractors, however, were slow to implement this agreement; after trade union pressure, the health minister was forced to write to chief executives appealing to them to "speed up implementation of the joint statement" (Warner 2006). This re-regulation was a reassertion of the strength of frontline staff and their unions. By fighting these private providers on the front line, to the point of threatening actual strike action, the frontline unions forced a change in national policy.

After working with the new employers under the PFI for several years, unions brought their concerns back to the government. By exerting pressure on the Labour Party, which was traditionally controlled and is still heavily influenced by the unions, the unions forced the adoption of a new policy that essentially guaranteed the end of the two-tier workforce. Although the change did not eliminate the PFI or remove private contractors, it ensured that privatized employees would be employed on broadly comparable terms and conditions. This caused some concern for PFI investors because one of the ways to extract profit from PFI schemes was to squeeze payroll costs; if payroll costs could not be cut, the potential profit would be more limited.

The paradox for trade unions was that national agreements on outsourcing and revised TUPE regulations provided some reassurance to transferred staff and facilitated the expansion of the private sector (Julius 2008). This made it more difficult for unions to oppose privatization when it was not obviously detrimental to the workers.

For workers and their unions, the real question was not whether private employers were worse than public sector employers but how to work with them. The unions had to maintain a two-pronged strategy. Although they opposed the PFI as a policy, they were unable to prevent it from happening in practice, so they had to learn to represent their members within the constraints of a PFI relationship. The priority became protecting members and potentially influencing and improving the PFI on a workplace-by-workplace basis. The GMB, for example, had national-level agreements with dozens of private sector companies that covered most of the major PFI service providers, and UNISON had agreements with a similar number (personal interviews, 2003). These agreements did not allow collective bargaining over wages, but they did cover some of the terms and conditions of employment. When the national agreement ending two-tier wages was combined with these bargaining agreements, the rights, protections, and voice of these private sector workers became quite similar to those of their public sector counterparts. Thus, although UNISON stood by its argument that the PFI is antithetical to the public service ethos, the ideological argument against outsourcing tended to be insufficient.

A Case in Point: Greenbelt

Stephen Bach and I selected for a case study the hospital for which I use the pseudonym of Greenbelt because it was fairly representative of the most successful PFI projects. When the interviews were performed, the hospital was fully operational and, unlike some other PFI hospitals, had not experienced major operational or financial problems. Greenbelt was built on the outskirts of a small city to replace a rather decrepit, long outdated building in town. It was opened early in the new millennium with nearly a thousand beds. The capital value was more than £150 million, and the PFI consortium included a number of construction and finance companies. The support services company, a major international player in the outsourced support services market, which I refer to here as Facilitiesco, had a 5 percent equity stake in the PFI consortium. The hospital buildings were owned by this private sector consortium, and the hospital effectively paid rent for the building and for support services provided by Facilitiesco on behalf of the consortium.

Greenbelt employed more than five thousand staff. Since the mid-1990s support services had been contracted out, so outsourcing of support services under the PFI did not represent a significant departure. Facilitiesco had not held any of the existing three- to five-year support service contracts in the trust. These contracts with a series of different contractors led to a proliferation of terms and conditions of employment and high staff turnover, which had resulted in falling trade union membership. Support staff working side by side were likely to be employed on completely different contracts, with different terms, conditions, and wages. This was a challenge for the unions. They shifted from representing workers under a single, national public employer with consistent pay and conditions and relatively low turnover to attempting to represent very low-wage workers with various terms and conditions under a fragmented set of private employers and consortia.

In hospitals that had strong local union branches, the unions tried to appoint separate representatives (known as stewards or convenors) to the direct public hospital employees and the privatized facilities staff. In the ideal situation, the representative(s) dealing with the private employer could press the company for improved pay and conditions and could develop expertise in the complex regulatory environment. At Greenbelt, the Facilitiesco union convenor (or chief steward/local president) highlighted the difficulties for the workforce and UNISON: "The MD [managing director of the subcontractor] came along, we invited him along for a day—we had lovely chats and everything else. Right at the crucial time of 'Look, will you be willing to sit down with us and get a recognition agreement where we can work together?' he leaned across the table and went 'I wouldn't have my mother-in-law tell me how to run my business. I certainly wouldn't have you'" (personal interview 2004).

Lay union officials had had negative experiences with previous contractors and contracting out, and this was important in evaluating the experience of Facilitiesco. Union activists were therefore skeptical about the position of the outsourced companies and whether they would be willing to work with the union at all. Initially, the private companies were not required to recognize the union or negotiate with it, so unions were dependent on attracting and retaining a strong enough membership to force the company to the bargaining table.

Facilitiesco derived 90 percent of its income from the public sector. It had become one of the most successful participants in the drive to marketize public services and was heavily dependent on this PFI to sustain its business model. It had grown rapidly, and in 2008 its turnover was more than £2 billion (Boxell 2009). These figures reflected Facilitiesco's track record of winning half the contracts it bid for, and it secured renewal of 90 percent of the contracts it held. All the main stakeholders we interviewed identified the importance of collaborative relations between the key parties. This enabled the Facilitiesco managers to work directly with Greenbelt managers without involving all the players in the PFI consortium. All members of the PFI consortium suggested that they were very selective about the contracts they bid for and that a key criterion was the attitude of the client (here, the hospital). Initially the PFI was a relatively unknown form of investment, so investors needed reassurance about the returns they could expect; an unsupportive client would increase the perceived risks. As a director of the investment company explained to me, "We like doing projects where the client is receptive to what we are providing; the ideal project is supportive client, supportive government, all parties are going into it to make it a success, and make it flexible and efficient. Unfortunately in life that is not always the case."

Facilitiesco managers expressed similar sentiments about the importance of a supportive client and how this affected their approach to employment relations. Facilitiesco stated that the Labour government's emphasis on partnership working had altered the climate in which outsourcing occurred and that they strongly preferred to gain union support before submitting a bid. Facilitiesco was willing to recognize trade unions at the local level on a contract-by-contract basis, although they were not willing to sign a national recognition agreement. This put the onus on local unions to show sufficient strength to force local recognition. Ironically, this approach may have encouraged strong local union organization, which was presumably not the intention of Facilitiesco. Although the company was opposed to national bargaining, this did not preclude national-level dialogue with trade unions. Facilitiesco's main focus was on ensuring that their track record was sufficient to gain workforce and local trade union support at the bid stage. As a manager explained, "The worst case is that if you don't get a tick [check] in the box from the local trade unions, all things being equal, you're not going to get the contract."

Many PFI companies initially granted unions recognition for bargaining over all issues except pay and benefits. Although the employer was willing to discuss certain issues with the union, pay negotiation was off the table. This allowed the contractors to claim that they were willing to work in partnership with, and negotiate with, unions while protecting their profits, usually at the expense of the wages of frontline staff.

The Consequences of the PFI in Greenbelt

Greenbelt opened on schedule with the support services workforce migrating over to Facilitiesco gradually as contracts came up for renewal. Facilitiesco employed approximately six hundred staff at Greenbelt for cleaning, portering, catering, car park management, maintenance, and grounds work. Of these, cleaning staff made up the largest group (about two hundred and fifty employees). Facilitiesco, however, had to manage a multi-tier workforce because staff had transferred from a number of different contractors; even within individual employers there was not absolute consistency. As the Facilitiesco manager emphasized, "The problems it causes—you know, two cleaners working alongside, they talk about how much they're getting: 'Why do you get that much, I don't get that much'—mayhem! Unmanageable, unnecessary things getting in the way of productivity."

To resolve this challenge, to address potential equal pay concerns, and to respect strong workforce traditions of unionization, Facilitiesco management agreed to recognize the main unions—Amicus, GMB, the Union of Construction, Allied Trades and Technicians (UCATT), and UNISON—and to provide full-time secondment to one of their employees, who had been a long-serving senior UNISON representative. One union representative was given a year of full-time release, which was subsequently extended, in order to work with Facilitiesco on a number of issues including the harmonization of terms and conditions of employment. This was especially important for Facilitiesco because it was increasingly difficult to justify variations in terms and conditions on equal pay grounds. There also were glaring gender inequities where jobs with similar skill levels were completely divided by gender: for example, the male employees in maintenance and parking were paid significantly more than the female employees in food service or cleaning. The disciplinary and grievance procedures of the former contractors also varied, and this reinforced the complexity of managing the workforce. As a union representative reported, "It was awful, Fred Bloggs had a disciplinary then you had to go through which disciplinary procedure you used for him because was he an ex-Mediguard or ex-initial or ex-RCO person? For our job as union people it was easier to simplify things, as it was for the company as well."

The strategy of the union at Greenbelt reflected the emphasis on a twin-track approach in which it engaged positively with the trust in identifying a preferred provider (contractor) and assisted Facilitiesco in harmonizing terms and conditions. But the union also threatened to strike on several occasions. The ability to threaten industrial action was dependent on high union membership. The Facilitiesco union representative recruited actively and increased the membership to four hundred out of a total of six hundred staff. Of this total, fewer than a quarter were originally NHS employees, and the remainder were recruited after the service had been outsourced. Staff saw Facilitiesco management in a more positive light than previous contractors because the managers were willing to adopt hospital policies and had a relatively positive attitude to training and development. Nonetheless, many of the lowest paid staff were paid at minimum-wage levels (£4.85 in 2004–5). This became a major issue in 2005 when UNISON submitted to twenty-four private contractors a national claim seeking the extension of NHS terms and conditions to all employees working on NHS contracts or as part of PFI arrangements. A substantial gap emerged between NHS and contractor rates.

Against a backdrop of national-level discussions, Facilitiesco made several offers in the range of £5.00 to £5.20 per hour, but these were not sufficient to gain the agreement of the workforce. In March 2005, UNISON members were balloted on an industrial action; after a turnout of 31 percent, 74 percent of the members voted for industrial action that would affect all support services at Greenbelt. During this period there was intensive lobbying by UNISON nationally and locally to encourage Facilitiesco to raise their offer.

One complication, noted in other studies of networks (Kinnie et al. 2005), was the difficulty of knowing precisely where pressure should be applied in the PFI consortium: Facilitiesco and Greenbelt both had an influence on the outcome. Pressure from the union was directed mainly at Greenbelt management, which wanted to avoid the political embarrassment of industrial action close to a national general election. Because the Labour government had staked significant political capital on improving and upgrading the NHS and its facilities, a strike could have had national political implications. As a trade union national officer explained, the branch chair's role was to "talk to the trust as well—'You don't want a strike do you?' If you are chief executive of a brand spanking new hospital . . . you don't want to be seen to be messing it up. [The branch chair] put pressure on the board of the trust, who put pressure on the consortium, who put pressure on Facilitiesco."

The trust board expressed its sympathy for Facilitiesco staff and suggested that all staff deserved "fair pay" but stopped short of endorsing the claim for parity with NHS employees. The dispute was resolved and industrial action averted after discussions mediated by the Advisory, Conciliation and Arbitration Service (ACAS), the national government arbitration service, which acted as a conduit for re-regulation and benchmarking between trusts by establishing an agreement that extended beyond Greenbelt.

In the case of Greenbelt, policy trickled up as a result of feedback. The union-led response to the bumpy implementation of the PFI led to a change in policy, specifically new protections for employees whose work was privatized. The discussions at ACAS formed the basis for national-level agreements between the trade unions, employers, and government that committed private contractors to migrate staff to NHS pay rates over time. Frontline staff used their workplace leverage to achieve better pay and conditions. Although the unions could not fight the PFI, they could ameliorate its impact. By initiating the pushback in the workplace, the unions were able to exploit the direct knowledge and experience of their members to achieve a positive outcome. It is worth noting that this frontline fight used traditional union strategies, focusing on negotiation backed with the threat of a strike. As a result of this dispute and the wider national-level agreement that followed, trade unions managed to attain substantial increases in terms and conditions of employment and to blunt the potentially detrimental consequences of marketization.

Extending Public Sector Standards in Greenbelt

The requirement to extend NHS pay to the Facilitiesco workforce demonstrated that government measures could extend public sector norms to the private sector. Union representatives at Greenbelt felt confident that, due to their ongoing pressure, negotiation, and monitoring, Facilitiesco staff were maintaining employment conditions similar to those that they had experienced when they were direct NHS employees. For example, Facilitiesco employees were able to access a variety of training programs. Cleaning staff were encouraged to undertake vocational credentialing courses offered by the British Institute of Cleaning Science. The Facilitiesco manager commented that "staff feel more motivated due to the national recognition that this award provides," and cleaning staff who achieved very high standards were given champion badges.

Many of the benefits for Facilitiesco staff were underpinned by the managerial and contractual inflexibility of the PFI contract. Because the detailed PFI contract spelled out the specific staffing requirements, Facilitiesco was bound to keep to its long-term commitment, regardless of the fluctuations of the market (or even changes in hospital needs). Because the trust was committed to payments to the consortium for thirty-five years irrespective of its changing needs, this provided more job security to the Facilitiesco staff than to the trust-based staff in an uncertain public expenditure context. Job security was tied to the length of the contract and although contracts were subject to market-testing or benchmarking every five to seven years, incumbent suppliers are in a strong position to retain the contract (National Audit Office 2007). By contrast, the high payments to the PFI consortium have contributed to financial difficulties and job insecurity for trust employees. This paradox was confirmed by the Facilitiesco representative: "The trust have started laying people off, several hundred they are looking at, and [Facilitiesco] have said we don't need to lay anyone off at all . . . so yes, people working with [Facilitiesco] have definitely got more job security than people working in the trust have."

An indication that NHS employment was no longer necessarily seen as more desirable than Facilitiesco employment was that in 2006 when the contract was up for renewal, unionized Facilitiesco staff expressed no interest in participating in an in-house (public sector) bid that if successful would have seen them transferred to NHS employment. This may have indicated a lack of ideological commitment to public employment, a general satisfaction with the new status quo, or both.

An Evolving System

Within the United Kingdom, regulation of outsourcing and PFI contracts is constantly evolving, particularly in response to pushback from frontline workers. The Labour government stated that it "only uses PFI where it can be shown to deliver value for money and does not come at the expense of employees' terms and conditions" (HM Treasury 2006, 4).

The government also established a number of codes of practice and standards that contractors have been required to implement. Although codes of practice represent informal executive regulation with uncertain consequences, trade unions have used the alternative dispute procedures (available to all employers and employees) to bring submissions to the government arbitration service, ACAS, to enforce these codes. In June 2009, ACAS found in favor of UNISON in its case against Parkwood Healthcare Ltd., which provides transport services to NHS trusts, because Parkwood was not complying with the code of practice (UNISON 2009b). This experience demonstrated that the codes of practice requiring comparable pay and conditions for privatized workers were legally enforceable—in this sense, the feedback loop was complete. The experience at the frontline forced a change in policy, through the work of the organized interests of the frontline providers.

The Labour government was highly interventionist in monitoring the standards that all hospitals and the contractors they employ must implement (for example, in relation to cleanliness). Finally there was extensive scrutiny of PFI contracts by the National Audit Office and parliamentary select committees, both of which placed large amounts of information about PPPs in the public domain (National Audit Office 2007; Public Accounts Committee 2007). Some of these reports received a good deal of media attention, for example, the highly critical report on the refinancing of the Norfolk and Norwich PFI hospital, in which the consortium of private investors accrued 71 percent of the gain (£82 million), which was viewed by some as an inappropriate outcome for the public sector (Public Accounts Committee 2006).

Greenbelt's experience resulted in complex outcomes for the frontline workforce in PFI hospitals, with employee concerns about the implementation of NHS terms and conditions and the uncertain status of trade union recognition set alongside attempts by Facilitiesco to invest in the workforce and to adhere to central government and NHS managers' requirements. These mixed outcomes arose partly from the contradictory combination of marketization, which increases provider competition and reduces the protection of public sector employment regulation, and partly from extending employment regulation to private providers as a way of limiting opposition to marketized reforms and enabling private sector service providers to develop some coherent employee management policies for their workforce.

The commitment of Greenbelt managers and the other PFI partners to working in partnership facilitated voice from frontline workers. This ultimately helped to improve the organization of frontline unions, which were able to parlay their influence from the workplace to the policy level. The evolution of PFI occurred in a context in which the Labour government was emphasizing the collaborative, mutually beneficial nature of public-private partnership, but this context was a necessary but not sufficient condition to promote new regulation, because the support of local PFI partners was crucial. At Greenbelt, the duration of the PFI contract was more than thirty years, and although support services are subject to periodic market testing by the PFI consortium, Facilitiesco had an equity stake in the consortium. While Greenbelt had not been immune to managerial turnover, many of the key union and managerial players had a long association with the trust and had established good working relationships. By contrast, many UNISON branch activists were less amenable to working with private sector employers, and these firms were often antagonistic toward trade unions (Bach and Givan 2008).

An effective workplace trade union organization at Greenbelt and some other hospitals, supported by national officers, enabled national agreements on the two-tier workforce to be implemented effectively at local level. This national agreement applied to all PFI workplaces, even those with weaker workplace union representation, less effective local leaders, or less receptive private sector partners. UNISON representatives at Greenbelt adopted an approach in which building workplace membership and securing support for industrial action was combined with positive engagement with Facilitiesco, locally and nationally. This approach generated development opportunities as well as pay increases for the UNISON membership. The involvement of ACAS also placed external pressure on the parties and reinforced a partnership-driven approach to employment relations that legitimated the equity and fairness concerns of the workforce, but also encouraged trade unions to commit to working within the new system.

In some other PFI hospitals with outsourced support services, however, trade union density was lower, and union organization was sparser. In these workplaces, union capacity to monitor and enforce forms of re-regulation was severely curtailed, and other tactics, such as working with nonlabor community organizations, could possibly be prescriptions for trade union strategy (Wills 2009). These less well-organized hospitals, however, benefitted from the change in national policy engendered by frontline unions at Greenbelt. The pushback and re-regulation essentially trickled up from Greenbelt and other similar hospitals into national policy and then back down to the less well-organized workplaces.

Since the early days of PFI, these deals have continued apace, albeit with the protected employment conditions created by this resistance from frontline workers and their unions. By the end of 2014 there were 728 current PFI projects (across all sectors) with a capital value of more than £55 billion (HM Treasury 2014). With the government taking on the financial risk of these projects, even as private investors reap profits that are essentially guaranteed, there has been no clear benefit to the public of the dependence on PFI projects for modernization of health service facilities (Pollock 2004; Pollock et al.

1997). As the physician and commentator Adam Gaffney observed, "By pushing costs decades down the road, however, [PFI contracts] left hospital trusts with poisonous obligations, later resulting in cuts in services and requiring government bailouts. In February 2012, for instance, the government bailed out some seven PFI-encumbered NHS trusts to the tune of £1.5 billion" (2014, 7).

Chapter 6

Building a Culture of Safety from the Front Line in the United States

Changes initiated by health care providers constantly take root in individual workplaces, but changes that trickle up from the workplace to the national level are less common. Chapter 5 showed an example of bottom-up change in the United Kingdom, and this chapter continues this theme with examples of bottom-up change initiated in hospitals in the United States. One of the strongest, broadest initiatives for change in health care organizations across the industrialized world has been the push to improve patient safety, clinical outcomes, and overall productivity. Theoretically at least, these changes might offer something to all the key stakeholders. If one assumes that provision of the highest quality clinical care is a universal priority, then these initiatives should be broadly appealing. In the best-case scenarios, administrators and policymakers suggest that certain performance enhancements can work as panaceas, producing more efficient (lower cost) health care with better clinical results.

Scores of books and articles have called attention to new advances in patient safety, many of which can be achieved at little or no cost (Agency for

Healthcare Research and Quality 2003; Gaffney, Harden, and Seddon 2005; Gordon, Buchanan, and Bretherton 2008; Gordon, Mendenhall, and O'Connor 2012; Koppel and Gordon 2012; Rogers et al. 2004; VitalSmarts 2008; Willett 2013; Woolf 2004). Different health care stakeholders may view this from slightly different angles; for example, staff may be wary of change introduced from outside the organization or of change that increases paperwork or is perceived to. Too often researchers have examined the effects of these programs on stakeholders in isolation from each other. How do these attempts to create and improve a culture of safety work in practice? How are they initiated and implemented? Do they work? And for whom?

Improving clinical care is at the heart of most efforts to improve health care. Although attempts to improve performance may include an array of objectives from reducing pain to increasing survival rates, reducing adverse events is always an important consideration. Of course, reduced errors should mean less pain, better survival rates, shorter hospital stays, and so on, but the relationship may not be straightforward or linear. Some of these errors may be so serious that the Joint Commission defines them as "never events" because they should never happen. The most extreme and shocking of these errors tend to be wrong-site surgeries (in which surgery is actually performed on the wrong place on the patient's body), but medication errors and preventable infections are also high on the list of avoidable mistakes (Michaels et al. 2007).

Although the issues of patient safety and provider safety are rarely examined together, frontline health care providers as well as patients are at risk, often due to poor safety procedures, pressure to save both time and money, and sometimes poor communication among employees. Research by the Joint Commission, one of the de facto US health care regulators, has emphasized that a hospital committed to creating a culture of safety cannot address patient safety and provider safety separately:

> Many health care organizations have "siloed" safety programs, creating one for patients, another for workers, and yet another for others who may be at risk. . . . What a loss! . . . The organizational culture, principles, methods, and tools for creating safety are the same, regardless of the population whose safety is the focus. . . . It is not possible to generate and maintain a culture of safety that encompasses only one or two of these groups. . . . A culture of safety—and the organization leaders who create and sustain it—will not be

considered legitimate and genuine if the culture excludes some groups within the organization. And, if an organization's culture of safety is not considered legitimate and genuine, it will not be valued and accepted—nor will it facilitate improved safety throughout the organization. (Joint Commission 2012a, vii)

As with so many attempts to change working life in hospitals, an effort to build bridges between silos tends to be easier said than done. It is remarkable that it took until 2012 for the Joint Commission to make this major statement on the importance of safety to all stakeholders, but it is not surprising given the emphasis by all interests, with the exception of unions, on patient safety alone. In this chapter I consider attempts, beginning in hospitals at the front lines of care, to create, implement, and diffuse a culture of safety for all who enter hospitals. I examine a range of different drivers of change, from the collaboration between physicians and patients (and their bereaved families) to reduce medical errors to the hard work by nurses' unions in forcing hospitals to take the safety of their employees seriously. Although there are numerous drivers of change in hospitals, from health insurance companies to private consultants who must generate their own work by proposing new practices about which they can advise, I focus here on the process of change that is initiated by hospital staff, from idea to implementation—or in some cases, nonimplementation.

The Front Line as a Resource

Frontline providers who identify both a problem and a solution and who understand the deep challenges of implementing this type of change have demonstrated that they can develop and promote successful initiatives. The resulting work processes exemplify new approaches initiated by health care workers on the front lines to improve patient care, provider safety, and overall hospital operations.

Sometimes, as in the case of the campaign for safe needles, workers and their unions fought for years to force hospital administrators and policymakers to take note and enact change. This policy change was completely reactive: hospital management never opted to use the safe needles, which are slightly more expensive than conventional needles, when they became available. Instead, the workers who were acquiring sometimes lethal diseases through the use of conventional needles organized their responses as bargained contracts and eventually in legislation. It is noteworthy not only that the change was initiated by frontline workers but also that most hospitals did not accept the change without being forced into it, primarily through change in US Occupational Safety and Health Administration (OSHA) regulations.

In other instances, hospital management actively solicited employee input and took action to create open workplaces by adopting processes to listen to employee voices and make continuous improvements. In some of these cases, midlevel managers played a key role in promoting and implementing changes that could be valuable for patients and employees alike (Hales and Pronovost 2006). It is worth noting, however, that the power structure in hospitals makes it much easier for physicians to implement changes (and indeed to rigorously evaluate these changes) than it is for any other frontline workers. Although physician-led changes have received a lot of media attention, in actuality the effect on the front line of the continuing emphasis on heroic doctors can be highly problematic (Koppel and Gordon 2012).

My argument here is not that change initiated by frontline workers is always right or successful, but rather that the knowledge and participation of frontline workers can be an essential catalyst in initiating and implementing change that benefits all the stakeholders in health care—patients, providers, and even payers. Recent evidence demonstrates that the health care delivery system is rife with perverse incentives, financial and otherwise, that may make improving patient care outcomes not advantageous for stakeholders. For example, a 2013 study showed that surgical complications increased the "hospital contribution margin"—in essence, the profit—for patient services and concluded that "many hospitals have the potential for adverse near-term financial consequences for decreasing postsurgical complications" (Eappen et al. 2013, 1599). Although complications lead to additional costs for hospitals, these costs are passed on to payers (specifically, Medicare and private insurers) at rates that generate a profit for the hospital.

Frontline workers are best positioned to understand the complex trade-offs in health care decisions and the ways in which stakeholder interests are not always compatible. The Joint Commission has begun to emphasize that "high reliability organizations"—its term for the safest hospitals—must have a safety culture that emphasizes both patient and staff safety and to recognize that the same tools, such as high trust and open communication, are necessary for both (Joint Commission 2012a). The Joint Commission is promoting the notion that there should not be trade-offs between patient and staff safety, or between a safety culture and cost, but rather that a comprehensive safety culture can reduce costs while improving outcomes for all. The key to the deep implementation of this culture, however, is the work and commitment of frontline staff.

Patient Safety

The founding moment in the patient-safety movement was the 2000 release by the Institute of Medicine of the report *To Err Is Human,* which documented the shocking number of fatalities in the United States because of medical errors of various kinds (Kohn, Corrigan, and Donaldson 2000). Particular horror stories sometimes gain media attention, such as the story of eighteen-month-old Josie King, who died in 2001 as a result of a central-line infection that she acquired in a hospital (Pronovost and Vohr 2010). King's family created a foundation dedicated to saving lives through improving patient safety, and her bereaved mother Sorrel has become a nationally known advocate on theses issues (Josie King Foundation 2007). A 2013 *New York Times* opinion piece recounted a medical error that led to the loss of the author's leg, and a near-fatal medication dosage error when the same author's wife was treated for blood clots (Southwick 2013). Both errors led to expensive medical treatment that should not have been needed as well as immeasurable pain and anguish resulting from preventable errors in hospitals. Stories such as Josie King's are everywhere in the patient-safety movement, illustrating the worst lapses of hospitals that result in tragic, usually avoidable complications and sometimes death.

Aligning with the physician's mantra of Do No Harm, patient safety has caught the imagination of patients and policymakers alike. As a result, policymakers, patients, family members, and health care practitioners have collaborated in pushing patient safety to the top of national agendas and promoting change on the front line. In 2004 the World Health Organization (WHO) created the World Alliance for Patient Safety in response to demand from its member countries. The WHO alliance was initially proposed by Sir Liam Donaldson, who was then the chief medical officer in the United Kingdom and a leading patient safety advocate; he has since become the WHO Envoy for Patient Safety.

Medical errors are costly in dollars as well as in lives. One study estimated the annual cost of hospital-acquired infections (the result of just one category of medical error or lack of care) to be potentially as high as $45 billion (Scott and Division of Healthcare Quality Promotion 2009). Hospital-acquired infections, which are frequently resistant to antibiotics, are a major concern. It seems everyone has a friend or family member who picked up a life-threatening infection in a hospital, often while there for a relatively minor procedure. Hospitals are dangerous places, as one newspaper account made clear: "Just ask Ruth Lepper, whose 74-year-old husband, Darwyn, had hip surgery in 2008 and died within months of complications from infections. Or Julie Rich, who is 69 and relies on an oxygen machine because of an infection she contracted after outpatient surgery. And Marcia Friedman, whose 91-year-old mother, Eleanor, was recovering from a blood clot when she got infected and died" (Allen and Richards 2010).

Unfortunately, *patient safety* is veering perilously close to becoming just another buzzword in the management and administration of hospitals. Every hospital now claims an emphasis on patient safety, and physicians writing in mainstream, nonspecialist publications such as the *New Yorker* have highlighted the problem of medical errors as well as possible solutions. Gawande, Pronovost, and others have demonstrated that the use of checklists, a safety feature borrowed from the aviation industry, can ensure that basic steps are followed and in the correct order. For example, providers have frequently been negligent in hand-washing (a key element in infection control), but checklists provided the simple nudge necessary to ensure complete compliance with hand-washing protocols in operating rooms (Gawande 2007, 2009a; Pronovost et al. 2006). The solutions (as popularized, although not necessarily as originally conceived) often focus on the technology of bedside care rather than the implementation of any new initiatives.[1] The reality of improving patient safety involves much more than photocopied or touchscreen checklists.

---

1. I use *technology* here following Kerr et al. (1964). In this sense, it refers to the structure and operations of the work tasks, not technology in the twenty-first century sense of denoting electronics and information technology.

The implementation of new work processes requires buy-in at every level of the workplace. This means that all frontline workers, not only doctors, will need a shared understanding of the problem, the cause of the problem, and the viability of the proposed solution. When staff do not believe the initiative will lead to any improvement in the quality of patient care, they are unlikely to implement the change. In the cases of checklists and hand-washing, the notion that a checklist was a quick fix that could be introduced by hospital administrators was a risky misinterpretation of the findings from their research; Pronovost and his collaborators carefully elaborate on why collaborative relationships and open communication are key to improving patient safety (Pronovost and Vohr 2010).

Worker Safety

We may think that the most dangerous workplaces in the United States are those with the most dramatic and sensational injuries, such as construction sites and oil rigs; however, according to OSHA, "more workers are injured in the health care and social assistance industry sector than any other" (US Occupational Safety and Health Administration 2008). The rate, as opposed to the absolute number, of injuries and illnesses is also quite high.

The safety of health care providers has never received as much attention as that of patients. In spite of the abundant health and safety risks for health care workers, the frequent problems of musculoskeletal injuries, stress, violence, and more tend to be ignored, in spite of the obvious link between these problems and turnover, both of which can in turn lead to worse clinical outcomes (Avgar, Givan, and Liu 2011a). Repetitive strain injuries and serious muscular problems (such as back pain) are not the result of accidents, and they do not tend to result in death, but they frequently build up over time and may ultimately disable a worker. Needlestick injuries expose frontline staff to a variety of dangerous blood-borne pathogens. Health care workers are also susceptible to hospital-acquired infections such as methicillin-resistant *Staphylococcus aureus,* although data on the prevalence of these infections are difficult to pin down (Allen and Richards 2010). In general, there has been little empirical research assessing how and whether patient and provider safety can be tackled in tandem, although many of the same strategies—communication, teamwork, and checklists, for example—seem apt for addressing both problems.

Although the problem is beginning to receive some government attention, action has been relatively limited. In November 2011, after the release of particularly worrisome US Bureau of Labor Statistics data on occupational illnesses and injuries for health care support workers, Dr. David Michaels, Assistant Secretary of Labor for OSHA, released a statement expressing his concern and the department's determination to take action:

> It is unacceptable that the workers who have dedicated their lives to caring for our loved ones when they are sick are the very same workers who face the highest risk of work-related injury and illness. These injuries can end up destroying a family's emotional and financial security. While workplace injuries, illnesses and fatalities take an enormous toll on this nation's economy—the toll on injured workers and their families is intolerable. . . . The workers that care for our loved ones deserve a safe workplace and OSHA is diligently working to make this happen. (Occupational Safety and Health Administration 2008)

In 2001, one of the Joint Commission's journals, the *Joint Commission Journal on Quality and Patient Safety,* published an issue focused on both patient and provider safety in which articles originally presented at conferences held in 1999 and 2000 examined the potential relationship between workplaces that are healthy for employees and the provision of high-quality health care. Several of the articles raised more questions than answers: for example, one article proposed frameworks from other industries that could be used to assess health care workplaces (Eisenberg, Bowman, and Foster 2001). For the most part, these articles identified major gaps in the existing literature and the need for more information. As Christine Kovner stated, "The primary problem is overall lack of research. When compared with biomedical research in areas such as cancer, symptom relief research such as that on incontinence, or health services research on areas such as access to care, research on staffing and patient/staff outcomes is meager" (Kovner 2001, 464–65). These researchers noted that although intuitively it seemed likely that workplaces that are safe and healthy for their employees are safer and healthier for patients, there was little empirical research that could confirm or refute this hunch.

Important agencies, such as the Agency for Healthcare Research and Quality (AHRQ), heeded this call and promised to fund further research. But the momentum died quickly, and the Quality Interagency Coordination Task Force, created by President Clinton in 1998 to encourage multiple government agencies to work together to improve patient safety (including through workplace safety initiatives), essentially died in 2000 (Agency for Healthcare Research and Quality 2000). This is deeply ironic, given that the seminal report *To Err Is Human,* which brought massive attention to the casualties of medical errors, was initially released in 1999, and it likely created a much greater space for research and action on these issues (Kohn, Corrigan, and Donaldson 2000). In the world of Washington policymaking, it is perhaps unsurprising that initiatives come and go and that priorities shift with the advent of a new presidency. But the rapid decline of federal interest in the safety of health care workers is particularly noteworthy because it coincided with the focus on patient safety following the release of *To Err Is Human* (Kohn, Corrigan, and Donaldson 2000). Most of the continued patient safety initiatives were then spearheaded by the AHRQ, but without a major focus on provider safety or the relationship between provider safety and patient safety (Agency for Healthcare Research and Quality 2003).

Workplace Safety Initiatives Graduating to State-Level Responses

Health care workers, particularly aides, orderlies, and those involved in moving patients, are at a very high risk of injury. The rate of musculoskeletal injuries, such as sprains and strains, for health workers is about three times higher than the rate of these injuries for construction laborers (US Occupational Safety and Health Administration 2013). Indeed, the Joint Commission noted that "few activities in health care link patient and worker safety more directly than lifting, transferring, repositioning, and ambulating patients" (Joint Commission 2012a, 62). As OSHA explains,

> These injuries are due in large part to overexertion related to repeated manual patient handling activities, often involving heavy manual lifting associated with transferring, and repositioning patients and working in extremely awkward postures. Some examples of patient handling tasks that may be

identified as high-risk include: transferring from toilet to chair, transferring from chair to bed, transferring from bathtub to chair, repositioning from side to side in bed, lifting a patient in bed, repositioning a patient in chair, or making a bed with a patient in it. (US Occupational Safety and Health Administration 2013)

It is important to note that many of these injuries are the result of repetitive movements, rather than of a single case of overexertion. Although the detrimental effects of poor patient handling are unlikely to be life-threatening for either patients or staff, such injuries tend to accumulate over time, and the effects are real, serious, and preventable: incorrect patient handling may eventually lead to an inability to work.

Health care workers are consistently forced out of their careers by such preventable injuries. Although lifts for patients are costly, the choice to do without them is also costly—in terms of injuries, nurse turnover, and early retirement, as well as in the possibility of litigation against employers. Bettye Shogren, a nurse from Minnesota, testified before a US Senate subcommittee about the career-ending injury sustained by her fellow nurse, Stacy Lundquist. Shogren read a statement from Lundquist, who was unable to be present at the hearing because of the severity of her injuries:

> I have had 4 surgeries over the last 3+years; I suffer from severe chronic pain which can only be controlled with medication. I can walk only short distances with a cane and must use a wheelchair when I leave my home. The pain is so intense that some days I think it would be better to be a paraplegic. I have lost my career. My injury fundamentally changed every part of my life. I can't walk, I can't drive, I can't shop, and I can't bike. I can't pitch a tent or camp or hike in the woods. I can't sleep or rest without medication and even then, I can't sleep very well. I couldn't pick up my first grandchild. I believe all of that could have been prevented if I had that piece of equipment. The pain I endure every day may never end. The rest of my life will never be what it could have been. (US Senate, Committee on Health, Education, Labor and Pensions, Subcommittee on Employment and Workplace Safety 2010)

Frontline workers in health care have high rates of musculoskeletal injuries because their jobs often demand lifting in awkward and improper ways. Safe patient handling (also known as zero lift or safe transfer) changes the physical set up of patient care so that patients are moved—often from one bed to another or from bed to chair—in a way that does not risk the patient's safety or the health of the caregiver. In safe handling, patients are moved safely and comfortably, without the risk of being dropped during a transfer, but the most crucial benefits of these improved procedures are to the front-line workers. Safe patient handling requires the use of a mechanical lift or hoist (often known by the brand name, Hoyer lift) to move patients, and to comply with the highest safety standards, a hospital must pay for the installation of these lifts and train employees in their proper use.

The campaign to protect health care workers from back injuries has moved between the workplace level and the state and federal levels (as was also the case with the campaign against needlestick injuries, to be discussed later). Many collective bargaining agreements include either a requirement for the use of patient lifts or a standing labor–management committee on safety (or similar) through which workers and management jointly determine best practices on workplace safety—and these practices almost inevitably include the use of lifts. In 2009, both the US Senate and House considered but did not enact the Nurse and Health Care Worker Protection Act. This act would have directed OSHA to revise its standards to require safe patient handling and injury prevention. In 2010, the Senate Subcommittee on Employment and Workplace Safety held hearings on the same topic, at which occupational health experts and nurses rehearsed the same arguments, but again no legislative action resulted, which was unsurprising given continued partisan paralysis in Congress at the time (Collins 2010). Arguments tended to focus on the high rate of injury to nurses and nursing aides and to link this with the ongoing shortage of nurses nationwide.

Since the 2009 act failed to gain traction, the major nursing unions have now focused attention on the state level, where unions continue to lobby for such legislation. Several states currently have safe patient handling legislation in place, and unions are pushing for the policy change in several others, including New York and Illinois (US Occupational Safety and Health Administration 2013). Legislation in other states is much weaker; for example, six states require health care workplaces to use safe handling practices, but other states simply promote safe handling, for example, through providing interest-free loans for health care organizations to purchase lifts. The state-level push is an example of unions using the available resources to protect all nurses. In unionized workplaces, safe lifting standards are often covered by the collective bargaining agreements, and unions have also deployed considerable resources to protect nonmembers. Again, this push has moved from the workplace, where bargaining primarily takes place with a single employer at a time, to state and federal campaigns designed to create a policy change that will ultimately cover all health care workers.

From Frontline Initiative to National Response

In addition to frontline initiatives for change moving up to the state level, there are also cases in which workplace challenges moved to the national level. Lorraine Thiebaud, a nurse and Service Employees International Union (SEIU) member, began campaigning for safer needles in her hospital, San Francisco General Hospital, in 1991. In 1992, Peggy Ferro (testifying as Jean Roe) told Congress about how she had contracted human immunodeficiency virus (HIV) from a conventional needle; in 1998, Ferro died of HIV. Congressional hearings were held again in 2000 (US House of Representatives 2000). It took almost a decade from these initial hearings for Congress to enact a law protecting workers from these preventable workplace accidents. Even as patient safety moved into the foreground in the media, provider safety was largely ignored. This may be because health care workers, especially nurses, have always suffered from high levels of workplace injuries, from violence to musculoskeletal injuries. Policymakers and health administrators seem to have been unable to make a link between the risks, injuries, and high level of burnout among health care workers and a subsequent shortage of these workers.

Historically, needlestick injuries have been a widespread problem in hospitals, and they have become particularly dangerous in an age of HIV and other blood-borne diseases. Not all needles are the same. Since the mid-1990s needle manufacturers have offered safety needles that make it almost impossible to stick something or someone accidentally. These needles are widely available, but they are more expensive than old-fashioned needles. Thiebaud began working with her SEIU local after several health care workers were infected with HIV and hepatitis through accidental needlesticks. The union local initially filed a grievance, which it supplemented with a petition as well as public posters and demonstrations. The union (in cooperation with the other unions in the hospital) eventually won the adoption of safety needles and formed a labor–management committee to prevent needlestick injuries (Thiebaud 2000).

After this initial success, the SEIU local worked to introduce the safety needles into other city hospitals and clinics. Thiebaud and others realized, however, that the problem of needlestick injuries was much broader and extended to all kinds of health workers and health workplaces. At this point, the campaign, which was aided by a series of investigative articles published in the *San Francisco Chronicle,* moved from San Francisco General Hospital to the state legislature in San Francisco. The SEIU began to lobby for a state-wide bill, an effort supported by Kaiser Permanente, a huge health care provider. The state law requiring safety needles was passed in 1998 and went into effect in 1999, but the battle was not over. Thiebaud and others turned their attention to national legislation. Thiebaud testified that health care workers felt safer with safety needles mandated by law and that employees should have this protection everywhere (Thiebaud 2000). Safety needles are more expensive, so it was important to make the case that the higher cost was a necessary investment in a safe work environment. Thiebaud testified that "SEIU and other health care unions, such as the American Federation of State, County and Municipal Employees, and the American Federation of Teachers, believe that the only truly effective way to prevent needlestick injuries nationwide is to pass a law requiring employers to evaluate and use safer devices." This was a logical strategy, given the patchiness of collective bargaining.

By 2000, a General Accounting Office (GAO) report examined the cost of needlestick injuries in hospitals, along with the possible costs and benefits of requiring the use of safety needles. The report acknowledged that the data available on needlestick injuries were quite poor. The GAO estimated that the use of safety needles would prevent 69,000 needlestick injuries a year in hospitals and would reduce exposure to HIV and hepatitis B and C (Heinrich 2000, 2). The report noted that a number of safety needles were available, although these devices varied in their features and efficacy. The GAO also stated that "there are obstacles to the use of needles with safety features, which include their increased purchase price compared with conventional devices, possible staff resistance to changes in the devices used, and the time required to train staff in the use of new devices" (Heinrich 2000, 5). The reference to "possible staff resistance" belittles both the extensive work front-line workers had already done to promote the use of safety needles and the risks staff were taking every day in using conventional needles. In fact, the major obstacle to the use of safety needles was the blanket long-term purchasing contracts that hospitals had with needle suppliers, which prohibited the hospitals from buying the safer needles because they were made by a different manufacturer than the one holding the contract (Blake 2010).

The Needlestick Safety and Prevention Act (2000) took effect in 2001 as an amendment to OSHA's Bloodborne Pathogens Standard. The new law gave all workers the protection that San Francisco General Hospital workers had won in their own workplace in 1992. This law required OSHA to issue revised standards about needle safety. The new OSHA standard required health care providers to use safer needles, needles that were slightly pricier than conventional needles but reduced the risk of accidental needlestick injuries, especially to health care workers. But it took more than a decade for the government to ensure the safety of all hospital workers (Blake 2010). The law was too late for Mary Magee (known only as Jane Doe until 2011), who was infected with HIV in 1987 through a needlestick injury (Allday 2011). And it was too late for scores of other health care workers who acquired diseases, and in some cases died, through these workplace accidents. The real tragedy of the situation is that even though these injuries are now preventable, they continue to occur.

Unions Leading Change from the Workplace

It is no accident that the most significant examples of changes initiated from the front line happened in unionized workplaces. Although unions are not the be-all and end-all of employee voice, it is generally true that workers who feel protected by a collective bargaining agreement are more likely to be comfortable speaking out about a problem or a promising idea. Whether changes trickle up through the grievance procedure, at the bargaining table, or through legislative lobbying, unions have a number of access points through which they can improve health care quality for both patients and providers. The most effective unions tend to be both agile and strategic. They are able to identify when a change might be achieved at the bargaining table and when campaigning for legislative or regulatory change might be more appropriate. This was true in my earlier examples of campaigns for safe needles and safer lifting equipment, but also true in the following case of the unit-based labor–management teams implemented at Kaiser, a massive, integrated health care system that operates primarily in the western states.

Kaiser Permanente's labor–management partnership demonstrates changes rooted in bargaining (Kochan et al. 2009), which may be the key site of wholesale change. What the participants refer to as the "partnership agreement" is a wide-ranging collective bargaining agreement. It covers all the usual areas, such as union security and grievances, but goes further to cover the mechanisms to initiate and implement improvements through joint work between labor and management. The partnership agreement itself essentially requires that new changes be introduced from the front line through a process of negotiation involving representatives of both labor and management. The shared labor-management objectives are summarized in the collective bargaining agreement: "By involving employees and unions in organizational decision making at every level, the Partnership is designed to improve the quality of health care, make Kaiser Permanente a better place to work, enhance Kaiser Permanente's competitive performance, provide employees with employment and income security and expand Kaiser Permanente's membership" (Kaiser Permanente and the Coalition of Kaiser Permanente Unions 2010).

The initial goal of the process was an ambitious shift to "an environment characterized by collaboration, inclusion and mutual trust." Among the many goals of the partnership are "creating a culture of safety" and a "comprehensive approach to safety." By including these areas in the partnership agreement, which is essentially a binding operating agreement like other collective bargaining agreements, managers and employees were bound to implement this strategic goal, and resources were available for implementation.

In this sense, then, the broader purpose of the arrangement was to foster employee voice and to create processes for frontline workers to take ownership of their work and play a central role in any changes. The rhetoric implies an end to top-down change.[2] The heart of the partnership is the construction of "unit based teams" who take charge of day-to-day operations, work envi-

---

2. The partnership did not include the California Nurses Association, a union philosophically and consistently opposed to labor–management partnership in all cases, which meant that 17,000 nurses in the partnership facilities were nonparticipants (Parks 2011).

ronment, improving performance, initiatives such as workplace safety, and work flows and design (Coalition of Kaiser Permanente Unions and Permanente 2011).

The Kaiser partnership is a blueprint for initiating change from the front line. Although the partnership itself was initiated not by frontline workers but by union leadership and management, the goal of the partnership was to institutionalize and mandate change from below. On the issue of workplace safety, the agreement states, "The Principles of Partnership will be used to engage frontline staff and supervisors in implementing the remedies that will eliminate hazards that cause injuries. It is recognized that in creating an effective culture of safety, alignment among all contributing Kaiser Permanente Departments must be achieved" (Kaiser Permanente and the Coalition of Kaiser Permanente Unions 2012, 40). The goal of eliminating workplace injuries is not an unusual one, but the commitment to do this through the engagement of frontline workers rather than through new policies pushed from the top-down is significantly different from most hospitals.

The move to partnership at Kaiser was an enormous task that required a wholesale shift from a culture where physicians and managers controlled much of the work to a flatter organizational structure with staff engagement at all levels. Traditional professional hierarchies and organizational silos make the creation of this level of employee control and voice a massive and costly challenge. Indeed, Kaiser's origins as a physician-led organization made a move to a flatter, less hierarchical organizational culture particularly challenging. Implementing a safety culture that encompassed both patient and staff safety was one of the many challenges tackled through this massive restructuring of the organization's entire decision-making process. The results of the partnership were very positive in terms of maintaining labor peace, but more difficult to quantify on other dimensions (Kochan et al. 2009). There were clear improvements through the partnership work in broad areas from health information technology to clinical outcomes, generally because of increased employee involvement (Kochan et al. 2009, 209).

In an analysis of the improved workplace safety outcomes achieved through the partnership, one study reported, "An articulated partnership process creates an environment in which frontline staff and management feel comfortable working collaboratively to overcome roadblocks to effective communication and workplace safety, along with other challenges. This mutual understanding and trust fosters a more respectful workplace and a problem-solving process that includes all voices" (Lazes, Figueroa, and Katz 2012, iv). About the effort to improve workplace safety, one area director observed that safety is "about building a culture of safety, learning and performance, and you can't have that unless everyone leaves work as safe and healthy as when they arrived. If the front line is not engaged in that process, it's not going to work. You can't assign the 'task' of workplace and patient safety. Everyone has to own these issues" (Willett 2013).

Implementing the partnership at Kaiser was expensive. The Office of Labor-Management Partnership had an annual budget of $16 million, and this reflected only the cost of the top-level implementation, not the time and other resources required within each unit. As Kochan and colleagues, who authored the definitive scholarly work on the Kaiser Partnership, put it, the partnership is a "success—but still a work in progress" (2009, 233). Indeed, ceding control over workplace change to workers on the front line is always going to be a complicated process.

Some within Kaiser have emphasized the partnership as an endeavor that has transformed Kaiser into a learning organization. This characterization emphasizes that ideas like continuous improvement are the major objective of the partnership, sidestepping the need for labor peace which was a major factor in the early days of the partnership. Schilling et al. (2011), who all hold senior positions within Kaiser, reflected on the partnership process as insiders in their analysis of the success of the Kaiser partnership in creating a learning organization with built-in mechanisms for continuous improvement. Their research sets forth a model that claims to account for both bottom-up and top-down change. They argue that each essential component of a learning organization requires both a top-down and a bottom-up strategy. These scholars suggest that successful changes will "engage the hearts and minds of frontline staff," which puts rather a sinister spin on the endeavor (Schilling et al. 2011, 533–34). Rather than empowering frontline staff to innovate and suggest new processes, the emphasis here is on making frontline staff feel involved enough that they will not resist any change imposed from above. Indeed, Schilling and his colleagues go on to demonstrate that implementation on the front line was extremely inconsistent; they acknowledge that when neither the frontline workers nor middle managers were consistently engaged in the process, the implementation remained uneven (Schilling et al. 2011, 539).

My conversations with Kaiser employees also revealed deeply inconsistent implementation, with some frontline managers continuing to operate as though the partnership did not exist, pushing policies without following the procedures mandated in the lengthy, written partnership agreement. Workplace safety was a key area of focus for many unit-based teams (who are required to meet for at least two hours per month), and successful implementation was built on both sensible safety precautions and the creation of an environment in which all staff in a unit felt comfortable speaking out about safety concerns. In San Diego, for example, workplace safety observation training was made available to all staff, rather than only to charge nurses and managers as had previously been the case (Lazes, Figueroa, and Katz 2012, 27). This expansion of communication lines and staff engagement, coupled with a flattening of the hierarchy, meant that front line staff were empowered to initiate remedies for problems in workplace safety.

Assessments of the success of the Kaiser partnership vary wildly. The core relationships at the center of the partnership have been complicated by upheaval within the union and a number of decertification and recertification votes. Nevertheless, it is clear that the partnership has been most successful where employee engagement has been deep and genuine and where frontline staff trusted that their suggestions and concerns were valued and were used to initiate change (Kochan et al. 2009; Lazes, Figueroa, and Katz 2012).

Fostering Frontline Feedback

The examples in this chapter, taken together, demonstrate that policy and practice are profoundly shaped by frontline relationships, which feed back to higher organizational levels and to the policy arena. The safe needle legislation is a telling example of successful change initiated at the front line, and it also demonstrates nurse-led change. Bottom-up change comes from all kinds of frontline workers, from nurses to janitorial staff, all of whom are well positioned to identify areas of improvement. In the hospital hierarchy, doctors traditionally hold all the power. As management in many hospitals has become highly professionalized, populated with more MBAs and fewer MDs, nurses have been sidelined and sometimes silenced in favor of career administrators as much as in favor of physicians. Even with an expanded administrative layer in hospitals, however, the providers of the actual patient care retain the ability both to initiate change and to thwart the implementation of policy they deem to be disadvantageous.

Frontline change may be initiated for any number of reasons—to save money, to improve patient care, or to increase employee safety among others. The health and safety of employees, particularly nurses, has never seemed to be a priority for hospital management. While on-the-job injury rates (particularly back injuries from lifting and other musculoskeletal injuries) have been extremely high in the United States and the United Kingdom, hospital management and national regulatory authorities have not made it a priority to improve employee health and safety. When and if frontline workers buy into the notion that a broad safety culture can improve a hospital both for its staff and its patients, they are more likely to see this as an important goal and work to further it.

Some research has shown that there is a relationship between good (beneficial) employment practices and improved patient care (see, for example, Avgar, Givan, and Liu 2011a, 2011b), but most often management prioritizes cutting costs and improving patient care and neglects the role of employees in bringing about any change. In the case of safe needle contract clauses and ultimately legislation, nurses and their unions were able to demonstrate that needlestick injuries were costly—even more costly than safety needles—so eliminating these injuries really was a shared interest for employees, administrators, and patients.

Some literature has criticized physicians for having egos that overshadow the role of others in the health care team, or at least the media portrayal of physicians, who putatively show great courage in innovating for improved patient care. Suzanne Gordon has criticized the notion of the heroic doctor who swoops in, identifies and addresses a problem, and then embarks on a whirlwind media tour, presumably for fun and profit (Gordon 2005). One example of such a figure might be Peter Pronovost, the pioneer of the use of checklists in surgery. Pronovost's work, widely promoted in the *New Yorker* by the writer-surgeon Atul Gawande, has demonstrated in fairly clear terms that the use of simple checklists can dramatically improve patient safety (Gawande 2007). Both Pronovost and Guwande maintain careers as frontline doctors, but they have also achieved national prominence and credibility that distinguishes them from the typical frontline physician. Pronovost's work, which uses data gathered from hospitals that have implemented checklists, has been hailed by some as a panacea for American health care, addressing the horrifying data on the risks inherent in receiving health care detailed in *To Err Is Human* (Kohn, Corrigan, and Donaldson 2000).

Media accounts have held up Pronovost as a visionary leader who has single-handedly created a safety culture in his hospital, crediting him with creating and implementing the checklist to reduce (and almost eliminate) dangerous central-line infections (Brody 2008). A closer look at Pronovost's work shows that, although others have given him a great deal of credit for his leadership in improving patient safety, his work consistently emphasizes the importance of flattening hierarchies and engaging all frontline employees in order to make positive changes (Pronovost and Vohr 2010). This essential aspect—the need for interprofessional collaboration for the successful implementation of this change—has been left out of much of the subsequent debate.

In their book explaining the use of checklists in improving patient safety, Pronovost himself, along with his coauthor Eric Vohr, consistently point to hospital culture as an obstacle to change. They discuss various aspects of relationships in hospitals (especially in the operating room) that might both make patients less safe and make it difficult to persuade these practitioners to change (Pronovost and Vohr 2010). For example, when nurses are afraid to question the actions of doctors, even when a safety protocol has been breached, patient care is at risk. When discussing how to change this culture, the authors emphasize the importance of empowering nurses to check the work of doctors and to challenge the physicians when they do not follow their checklists. They tend to use the notion of culture as shorthand for the complex and sometimes toxic relationships that are common in hospitals, where hierarchies are often strictly enforced by those at the top (the physicians) and where this power dynamic conditions all interactions. Pronovost and Vohr make clear that nurses, in particular, must be given the confidence to speak up when they see a problem and the knowledge that they will not be humiliated or scolded by doctors and that they will not face punishment for daring to disagree with a doctor. The same hesitancies can also be a problem with junior and senior physicians and, indeed, between doctors with different specialties. They contend that problems like these often manifest themselves in "poor communication," which in turn is blamed for medical errors, but they also make clear that this poor communication comes from a flawed system, a dysfunctional workplace culture (Pronovost and Vohr 2010).

Crucially, one of the key aspects of the success of the checklist strategy is allowing, and even encouraging, nurses to intervene when doctors do not use the checklist or do not correctly follow each step. It is remarkable that hospital policies have had to specifically state that nurses can question doctors, and this speaks to the strict, longstanding hierarchy in hospitals, and perhaps most of all in operating rooms, which results in the view that a nurse questioning the judgment or practice of a doctor is a form of insubordination. The titles of books on nursing reveal the lack of voice that nurses have always experienced in the workplace, such as *From Silence to Voice* (Buresh and Gordon 2006) and *Say Little, Do Much* (Nelson 2001). Many of the most successful advances toward creating a safety culture in hospitals have emphasized empowering all frontline workers to speak out as advocates for their patients and themselves, even when contradicting physicians.

In this push to create an environment where employees are comfortable voicing concerns, some hospitals have embarked on formal programs to address a climate that might deter workers from coming forward. After Maimonides Medical Center in Brooklyn initiated programs to increase "mutual respect" and reduce conflict, they were particularly proud of empowering nurses and other staff to voice their concerns to doctors without fear of reprisal (Givan 2010–11). In an interview, a Maimonides employee gave a specific example of a nurse speaking up in surgery to query a possible problem, and this interviewee pointed out that the newly implemented multifaceted conflict-management system had allowed the nurse to speak up. In some sense, the conflict-management system leveled the traditional hospital hierarchy (see also Givan 2010–11).

One of the new systems implemented at Maimonides hospital, the hospital-wide code of mutual respect, was an extension to the whole hospital community of an earlier code that had applied only to doctors. The importance of physicians treating each other with respect is obvious, but physicians rarely work in isolation from other hospital staff, and it is clear that requiring respect among physicians alone is only a partial solution when there is an atmosphere lacking in respect or civility. As one of the leaders in implementing and broadening the code put it, there was a problem with poor communication, and hospital leadership was aware that this could have a negative impact on patient safety (VitalSmarts 2008). My conversations with hospital leaders, however, made it clear that their concern was not only patient safety but also employee relationships and satisfaction. As my own workplace interviews and published accounts of the implementation of the code make clear, nurses were particularly grateful for this specific and explicit form of empowerment (personal interviews 2009; VitalSmarts 2008). The Maimonides experience underscores the link between the empowerment of frontline staff and patient care outcomes.

These examples demonstrate the importance of giving voice to workers on the front line, but the question of how these programs are actually implemented remains. For example, any hospital can state that all staff have the right to speak up when they see a problem, but actually creating a culture of empowerment and voice is more challenging than creating a written policy. In successful examples, such as that of Maimonides, frontline staff were crucial in implementing the new policy and in developing the code. Indeed, through mechanisms similar to the unit-based teams at Kaiser Permanente, Maimonides devoted significant staff resources to ensuring that partnership means the genuine engagement of frontline workers (Lazes, Figueroa, and Katz 2012).

Indeed, even the lead advocate for checklists, Peter Pronovost, coauthored an article pointing out that perhaps the media frenzy over checklists and their miraculous effects was overblown (Bosk et al. 2009). "Reality Check for Checklists" was a response to widespread misinterpretation of the research on the successful use of checklists in improving patient safety. These authors pointed out that "the mistake of the 'simple checklist' story is in the assumption that a technical solution (checklists) can solve an adaptive (sociocultural) problem." They observe that the real success of checklists was in their implementation—or, as they put it, "how support was mobilized for coordinating work around infection control" (Bosk et al. 2009). It was not the new protocol that was noteworthy but rather the mechanism for obtaining broad support from the staff responsible for implementing this protocol. The authors explained how the new protocol created social networks and allowed nurses and physicians to jointly lead implementation teams. In fact, their article serves as a corrective to the view that checklists or physicians can, in isolation, improve patient safety. Rather, Bosk and colleagues characterize this experience as a story of communication, frontline empowerment, and teamwork:

[the successful use of checklists to improve patient safety] was achieved by allowing teams to customize the implementation of evidence locally, and challenging assumptions about who has relevant knowledge, who counts as an expert, and who is able and ought to act to improve safety. Indeed, it would be a mistake to say there was one "Keystone checklist": there was not a uniform instrument, but rather, more than 100 versions. Each ICU, informed by evidence and a prototype, was encouraged to develop their own checklist to fit their unique barriers and culture. Taken together, what the Keystone programme did was change workers' motives for cooperating so that they internalised new norms: the new way became taken for granted as "the way we do things around here." (Bosk et al. 2009)

There have been other attempts to improve patient safety, with successful outcomes closely linked to the engagement of frontline employees. In one effort to reduce central-line infections, providers in Pennsylvania attempted to use lean production methods to leverage the tacit knowledge of frontline staff for improved patient safety and reduced infections (Shannon et al. 2006). The use of these lean techniques, derived from the so-called Toyota model of production (see Womack, Jones, and Roos 1991), does not fit perfectly into either the top-down or bottom-up category of change implementation. The decision to move to the continuous improvement model is almost always taken by top hospital administration, but this model does not function without the cooperation of frontline staff. As with Pronovost's checklist, Shannon's team focused on empowering staff to both understand and question the appropriate processes. Their solution involved significant improvements both in training for frontline staff and in the actual methods used to place central-line catheters, for example, in the introduction of anti-microbial dressings.

These new processes were identified by a collaborative team made up of doctors and nurses who were responsible for placing central-line catheters in patients. By allowing the frontline staff to both identify the key problems and create a solution, the hospital created a new process with the buy-in of those who had to implement it. According to Shannon and colleagues, the changes were not easy to implement on top of an embedded hierarchical hospital culture, because of "the continuous struggle between standardizing practice and the fierce adherence to physician autonomy that constitutes a significant barrier to patient safety efforts in organized medicine" (Shannon et al. 2006, 485). These authors reported a significant decrease in mortality from central-line infections within a year of implementing the new procedures (Shannon et al. 2006).

These changes were initiated from the front line and were implemented through a slow and inclusive process. What was important was not what the changes were, or indeed what frontline workers initially thought of the new procedure, but the mode of implementation: intensive staff dialogue and the inclusion of all relevant workers. These changes had several important attributes in common: They were initiated by workers, based on their own knowledge of their jobs, and they responded to legitimate problems and avoided the whiff of change for its own sake. In this sense, they deployed the lean production concept of continuous improvement, exploiting the expertise of those who actually carried out the work. But these changes were not technological changes. They were changes that required buy-in and cooperation from workers, sometimes in ways that challenged their traditional views of their work.

Indeed, other recent studies have begun to emphasize teamwork as crucial in the improvement of clinical outcomes (Avgar, Givan, and Liu 2011a; Gittell 2009; Gittell et al. 2000). As one study puts it, "To achieve the best possible outcomes, the work of the multidisciplinary team must be coordinated and orchestrated in a seamless, supportive manner. . . . A leader can promote collaborative work, mutual worker support, goal-directed behavior, positive team perceptions of performance, and efficient resource utilization" (Green 2007, 587). It is clear that the role of the leader (in some cases, a physician) is crucial, but the key roles for this leader are facilitating cooperation and communication.

Maimonides hospital offers similar examples of effective workplace unionism engaging frontline workers and creating opportunities for frontline workers to question current practices and initiate changes, regardless of their places in the traditional hierarchy. For several years, hospital management engaged with the union in an intensive partnership program, where each side worked to open communication in order to improve hospital performance. This deepening of the workplace dialogue occurred in the context of well-established collective bargaining. As in the British Greenbelt case, the success of the partnership, as reported by key participants, rested on particular individual attributes, particularly on those of union representatives. This partnership is ongoing, but it has already resulted in measurable performance improvement. The success stories so far include the introduction of a highly responsive conflict resolution system and the reduction of the time it takes the ward staff to respond to bedside alarms. It is clear that without the open dialogue and the sincere buy-in from both management and the union, these new programs could not have been successfully implemented. The success of these joint efforts also highlights the fact that the union was focused on improved performance for all the hospital stakeholders, rather than on imagined, antiquated expectations of protection and job control.

Workplace issues can filter up beyond bargaining and into national precedent and legislation. As with the example of needle safety, the battle for minimum nurse–patient ratios emerged from a workplace problem. As the nursing shortage intensified in the 1990s, hospitals were relying on automated "acuity" systems that used software to determine, on the basis of the severity of the particular caseload on a floor, how many nurses were needed at any particular time. Nurses believed that these automated algorithms did not always allow for sufficient staffing and began to campaign, through either multiemployer bargaining or at the legislature, for regulatory change (Gordon, Buchanan, and Bretherton 2008). Like the needlestick prevention laws, this institutional change stemmed from the workplace and was driven by the common workplace experiences of bedside nurses.

The cases I report in this chapter document that real change can and does emanate from the front line, and the route to successful change, especially in the creation of a safety culture in hospitals, is from the front line to the higher levels of policy. Even good ideas will fail if they do not engage and empower health care workers on the front line and create openings for employee voice that run counter to centuries-long workplace hierarchies. Eventually, many of the most successful ideas produce instructive empirical data and forceful solutions, such as the clear reduction in needlestick injuries in hospitals using safe needles, that can lead to changes in national policy. These policies can spread most effectively when frontline workers share their experiences with legislators and regulators, leading to the broader diffusion of changes initiated at the workplace.

Chapter 7

From the Health Care Workplace to the Health Care System

Learning from the United States and the United Kingdom

To look ahead to future changes in the Anglo-American health care systems, this chapter resituates in their national contexts the cases I have discussed in earlier chapters. In both the United Kingdom and the United States there are ongoing changes in the areas of accountability, central regulation, privatization and resistance, and the still-growing safety movement. The constant flood of changes in the health care system in both countries is unlikely to change. Rather, changes will keep coming, and most of them will be initiated and imposed from above, by regulators and policymakers with little understanding of frontline work. The cases I have detailed illustrate how and when more appropriate changes can occur. The most optimistic reading would suggest that if we listen to frontline workers we can make lasting changes for the benefit of everyone—patients, providers, and payers. Maintaining safe staffing levels is perhaps the clearest example of this kind of change, yet in spite of its proven success in improving health outcomes and working conditions, few governments are willing to pass minimum nurse–patient ratios into law.

In all too many cases where change is needed there is little or no organizational learning. Those with the power to create policy or protocol are primarily interested in maintaining this power rather than learning from experience and helping hospitals positively evolve. In spite of the constant onslaught of new initiatives designed to improve health care, save money, or both, the delivery of care is not improving, and intractable problems remain. These problems include burnout of frontline staff, perverse incentives, and wrong-headed accountability schemes, and the solutions are not to be found by policymakers who are capable only of seeing the problems from 30,000 feet. The cases I have investigated have shown that when employees are engaged in solving the problems that affect them most directly, workable, realistic, and incremental solutions can and do emerge. When frontline workers act as an organized interest group, they can initiate and implement changes that make a lasting difference. Those who wish to improve patient care outcomes should be mindful of this and avoid adopting the latest fad from someone who has rarely set foot in a hospital. The quest for new practices that benefit all stakeholders can continue only if administrators and regulators prioritize improving the workplace for employees, not only for patients or for the sake of the bottom line (Givan, Avgar, and Liu 2010).

The Health Care Workplace Illuminates the Realities of the Health Care System

An integrated analysis of the employment relationship in the workplace within the larger policy issues that concern health sector employment—such as the discussion of the relationship between the Joint Commission's focus on patient safety and actual practices in the workplace—pushes our understanding much farther. By covering both the policymaking and the policy implementation stages, the conceptual framework I offer here creates a broader understanding of the true veto points in the process of health care restructuring.

Much research on employment relations focuses either on the workplace level or on the national political level. Although interviews with employees and managers can create strong arguments about the role of union representatives, the views of staff, and the relationship between management and employees, these interviews often fail to capture key macroeconomic and political issues that affect workplace relationships, such as the ways in which policy decisions create and influence these workplace relationships (Cully et al. 1999; Fairbrother 1996; Heaton, Mason, and Morgan 2002; Piore and Sabel 1984; Waddington and Kerr 1999). Similarly, works focusing on political institutions often miss the key steps between policy creation and policy implementation, and they do not fully comprehend the power dynamic in the workplace itself (Anderson and Mann 1997; Daley and Howell 1992–93; Monbiot 2000; Panitch and Leys 1997). Green-Pedersen and Haverland argue that most research on welfare focuses on either the national level or the sectoral level, and that "the national and sectoral level must be connected" (2002, 48; see also Moran 2000). In line with this suggestion, researchers must take their proposed research agenda farther by also examining the dynamics within the workplaces of the health care system, while bridging the workplace and the policymaking arenas. The framework used to analyze the cases in the previous chapters is based on the complex dynamics between as well as within these two levels of analysis.

I have argued that there is an underlying Anglo-American model of health care delivery, even though the systems are quite different in terms of payment and ownership. The Anglo-American model is characterized by the legacy of the professional power of physicians, which structures both the primary and acute care sectors. In both countries, there are key trends toward greater accountability and monitoring, higher quality care, privatization and competition with a strong current of resistance, and centralization of regulation.

Locating the Similarities amid the Differences

In health care workplaces, the dynamics on both sides of the Atlantic bear more than a passing resemblance. One key explanation for the enduring similarities across countries is the dominance of professional roles and the hierarchies that structure hospitals; these organizations operate within similar parameters and constraints in each country. As the examples of the Healthcare Commission in the United Kingdom and the Joint Commission in the United States have illustrated, targets and performance standards cannot simply be imposed from above. Rather, the workplace dynamic determines whether and how these standards are implemented.

Hospital managers in both countries face the constant challenge of asking professionals to change the way they work. Hospital organizations in both countries are structured around a professional hierarchy, with entry into the professions controlled by powerful professional organizations (see also Kleiner 2006). In a hospital in either country, one can observe a workforce stratified by professional and occupational groups. In many cases, professionals are managed only by members of the same profession: doctors manage doctors, nurses manage nurses, social workers manage social workers. The relationships between these groups, each with its own credentials, qualifications, and experience, are the foundation of the broader workplace relationship in both countries. The overlay of the bureaucratic structure on this professional structure makes it difficult for any hospital to implement quick or drastic change.

The comparison, then, within the Anglo-American model tells us where this model truly contains commonalities and where specific institutions, ownership, and finances make differences that are truly consequential. Practitioners in each country can and should learn from the comparison; both the similarities and the differences are instructive and illuminating.

Looking Ahead

In the United Kingdom, David Cameron's Conservative Party explicitly campaigned on a platform of ending top-down change in the National Health Service (NHS), claiming, "We will stop the top-down reorganizations and pointless structural upheavals that have done so much damage in the NHS," and "With the Conservatives there will be no more of the tiresome, meddlesome, top-down restructures that have dominated the last decade of the NHS" (Cameron 2008; Eaton 2013). Cameron's coalition government went on to pass the 2012 Health and Social Care Act, variously described as "the most controversial piece of NHS legislation in more than two decades," "the biggest top-down reorganization of the service in its history," and "the most egregious act of vandalism against the people of England" (Eaton 2013; Pollock 2015; Timmins 2012). This act shifted the power center of the NHS to local primary care groups who were responsible for "purchasing" all services for their patients.

National leaders are willing to rhetorically embrace the notion that top-down change is often unsuccessful. This rhetoric, however, tends to belie a continued dependence on high-level actors who propose changes without seeking the input and insights of frontline workers. Simon Stevens, a Briton who started his career in the NHS and spent over a decade as an executive in the American health care giant UnitedHealth Group, eventually returned to the United Kingdom as the chief executive of NHS England. The political commentator Polly Toynbee observed when Stevens took on his new role for the Conservative government that "Stevens will find many perversities in the competition culture. He said top-down control was a disaster—but he may find fragmentation and lack of strategic control far worse" (Toynbee 2013).

Earlier in his career, while working as a health policy adviser for Tony Blair, Stevens, critiquing the role of physicians in the NHS, had said that the "top-down challenge is therefore likely to have an ongoing place in the English health reform pantheon" (Stevens 2004). As the chief executive of the NHS in England under the Cameron government, Stevens changed his tune: "We call on the next government not to introduce any further top-down administrative reorganizations . . . There is no right answer as to how various bits of the NHS administration are organized but there's a wrong answer, and that's to keep changing your mind. That's what we don't want" (Riley-Smith 2014). This statement was rather bold, given that the government that had appointed Stevens had introduced one of the largest top-down changes the NHS had seen in decades. Stevens also made this claim at a time when austerity cuts and the new purchasing structures of the 2012 Health and Social Care Act were stretching the health service to its limits and forcing providers to rely on contracting out services. Sir David Nicholson, the NHS England chief executive who had preceded Stevens, had described the changes in the Health and Social Care Act as "a reorganization so big you can see it from outer space" (Cameron 2014).

The fear in the United Kingdom of the NHS becoming marketized to the point of resembling the US system continued with the election of the Conservative government (outright, without the need for coalition partners) in 2015. A symbolic bill with no chance of success was introduced to parliament calling for the end of private contracting and the "reinstatement" of the NHS. It claimed that "US healthcare 'solutions' are the death knell for the NHS. The NHS must be reinstated and 25 years of pernicious marketization reversed" (Pollock and Roderick 2015).

Assuming a future government does not undo the Obamacare legislation in the United States, one can expect an ongoing reliance on publicly purchased health care, which even in a fully marketized system is a key example of resistance to neoliberalism. Some analysts suggest that employer-purchased health insurance will decline as more employers will choose not to offer coverage and their employees will purchase their insurance on the exchanges (Emanuel 2014). The Affordable Care Act and its attendant regulatory changes affirmed requirements for performance monitoring and a reliance on data collection for everything from the Medicaid Delivery System Reform Incentive Payment Program (DSRIP) to the much vaunted comparative effectiveness research program for determining treatment protocols and public health priorities (Donnelly 2010; Gates, Rudowitz, and Guyer 2014).

Marketization creates fragmentation, but top-down changes still dominate when centralized regulation and ongoing programs of monitoring and accountability dominate the systems. The degree of future privatization and competition in each country remains somewhat unknown, but the reliance on individual pioneers or top-down strategies produced by consultants will continue, and implementation through the pathways of centralized regulation and centralized monitoring will continue. One can only hope that change from the front line will also be allowed to continue.

Indeed, in both countries there are signs of ongoing change initiatives coming from frontline workers and their organizations. In many states as well as on the federal level there are strong safe-staffing movements trying to implement the same minimum nurse–patient ratios that have been successful in California (National Nurses United 2015). In the United Kingdom, an incremental move toward monitoring staffing levels (rather than implementing minimum ratios) was put on hold by the newly empowered Conservative government in 2015, much to the chagrin of both UNISON and the Royal College of Nursing (Merrifield 2015). Both major UK unions representing nurses continue to emphasize this issue and to fight for minimum ratios that ensure high-quality care. Similarly, in the United States various campaigns focused on safe patient handling or "zero lifts" to reduce musculoskeletal injuries for nurses have taken root. As of this writing, ten states have passed some protective legislation in this area, and the movement is still working to reduce the horrific levels of life-changing injuries that continue to affect the nursing workforce (Zwerdling 2015).

As I hope this book has made clear, there is no panacea; literally, there is no cure-all for the problems in the health care system. Just as there is no cure-all, there is no perfect health care system. All systems contain trade-offs, priorities, and compromises. The workings of a system and of an individual hospital result from very human decisions, taken within a framework of regulatory and resource constraints. I have tried to argue not that bottom-up change is always better than top-down change, but that employee engagement is essential, no matter where the change is initiated.

As Robert Wachter, a prominent US physician, commentator, and patient-safety advocate noted, the NHS might seem to be set up for effective top-down interventions, and he has argued that the fragmentation of the US system makes broad change quite difficult. However, after he had spent a sabbatical in the United Kingdom, learning about the workings of the NHS, he observed:

> Before I arrived here, I assumed that the UK had a major advantage when it came to improving patient safety and quality. After all, a single-payer system means less chaos and fragmentation—one payer, one regulator; no muss, no fuss. But this can be more curse than blessing, because it creates a tendency to favor top-down solutions that—as we keep learning in patient safety—simply don't work very well. . . . The bottom line from analyses of complex systems is that over-managing workers through boatloads of top-down, prescriptive rules and directives may be more unsafe than tolerating some degree of flexibility and experimentation on the front lines. (Wachter 2011)

Again and again, those who observe both systems see profound advantages and disadvantages in each country. What they have in common, crucially, is that each system is in a state of constant evolution, and the stakeholders have some influence over the direction and form of future changes.

The trends of increased accountability, strong centralized regulation (sometimes captured by private interests), neoliberalism and resistance, and the push to improve quality are all working on the Anglo-American model at the same time, although not necessarily in the same direction. The cases I have investigated reveal that change from above without strong employee engagement is a difficult path to improvement, often fraught with perverse incentives and unintended consequences. Although employee-led change may not be the only route to improved health care quality, it provides a clearer path to evidence-based changes that work for both patients and health care providers.

References

Abramowitz, Michael. 1991. "On the Road with a Hospital Inspector." *Washington Post,* August 27, 1991. https://www.washingtonpost.com/archive/lifestyle/wellness/1991/08/27/on-the-road-with-a-hospital-inspector/cee4d4ed-8c69-407e-8598-e64189431b45/.

Accreditation Council for Graduate Medical Education. 2010. DIO News: Institutional Review. http://www.acgme.org/acgmeweb/Portals/0/DIO_News_Apr10.pdf.

AFL-CIO. 2007. California Nurses Association/National Nurses Organizing Committee Joins AFL-CIO. http://www.aflcio.org/Press-Room/Press-Releases/California-Nurses-Association-National-Nurses-Orga.

Agency for Healthcare Research and Quality (AHRQ). 2000. "Archive: About QuIC." Quality Interagency Coordination (QuIC) Task Force. http://archive.ahrq.gov/quic/about/index.htm.

———. 2003. "Chapter 3. AHRQ's Patient Safety Initiative: Breadth and Depth for Sustainable Improvements." In *AHRQ's Patient Safety Initiative: Building Foundations, Reducing Risk. Interim Report to the Senate Committee on Appropriations.* Publication 04-RG005. Agency for Healthcare Research and Quality, Rockville, MD. http://www.ahrq.gov/qual/pscongrpt/psini3.htm.

Aiken, L. H., S. P. Clarke, and D. M. Sloane. 2002. "Hospital Staffing, Organization, and Quality of Care: Cross-National Findings." *International Journal for Quality in Health Care* 14 (1): 5–13.

Aiken, L. H., S. P. Clarke, D. M. Sloane, J. Sochalski, and J. H. Silber. 2002. "Hospital Nurse Staffing and Patient Mortality, Nurse Burnout, and Job Dissatisfaction." *Journal of the American Medical Association* 288 (16): 1987–93.

Allday, Erin. 2011. "Nurse Who Contracted HIV with Jab Sheds Anonymity." *San Francisco Chronicle*, December 10, 2011. http://www.sfgate.com/news/article/Nurse-who-contracted-HIV-with-jab-sheds-anonymity-2394068.php.

Allen, Marshall, and Alex Richards. 2010. "A Hidden Epidemic." *Las Vegas Sun*, August 8, 2010. http://www.lasvegassun.com/news/2010/aug/08/hidden-epidemic/.

America's Health Insurance Plans. 2010. "Who We Are." http://www.ahip.org/content/default.aspx?bc=31%7C42.

American College of Surgeons. 1919. "The Minimum Standard." Posted May 25, 2006. http://www.facs.org/archives/minimumhighlight.html.

American Nurses Credentialing Center. 2014. "History of the Magnet Program." American Nurses Association. http://www.nursecredentialing.org/magnet/program overview/historyofthemagnetprogram.

Anderson, Paul, and Nyta Mann. 1997. *Safety First: The Making of New Labour.* London: Granta.

Ash, Michael, and Jean Ann Seago. 2004. "The Effect of Registered Nurses' Unions on Heart Attack Mortality." *Industrial and Labor Relations Review* 57 (3): 422–42.

Audit Commission. 1999. *A Measure of Success: Setting and Monitoring Local Performance Targets.* London: Audit Commission.

——. 2000. *On Target: The Practice of Performance Indicators.* London: Audit Commission.

——. 2003. *Targets in the Public Sector.* London: Audit Commission.

——. 2012. *By Definition: Improving Data Definitions and Their Use by the NHS.* Audit Commission.

Avgar, Ariel C., Rebecca K. Givan, and Mingwei Liu. 2011a. "Patient-Centered but Employee Delivered: Patient Care Innovation, Turnover, and Organizational Outcomes in Hospitals." *Industrial and Labor Relations Review* 64 (3): 423–40.

——. 2011b. "A Balancing Act: Work–Life Balance and Multiple Stakeholder Outcomes in Hospitals." *British Journal of Industrial Relations* 49 (4): 717–41.

Bach, Stephen. 1999. "Personnel Managers: Managing to Change?" In *Employee Relations in the Public Services: Themes and Issues*, edited by Susan Corby and Geoff White, 177–98. London: Routledge.

Bach, Stephen, and Rebecca Kolins Givan. 2010. "Regulating Employment Conditions in a Hospital Network: The Case of the Private Finance Initiative." *Human Resource Management Journal* 20 (4): 424–39.

Bach, Stephen, Rebecca Kolins Givan, and John Forth. 2009. "The Public Sector in Transition." In *The Evolution of the Modern Workplace*, edited by William Brown, Alex Bryson, John Forth, and Keith Whitfield, 307–31. Cambridge: Cambridge University Press.

Bach, Stephen, Ian Kessler, and Paul Heron. 2008. "Role Redesign in a Modernised NHS: The Case of Health Care Assistants." *Human Resource Management Journal* 18 (2): 171–87.

Berenholtz, S. M., P. J. Pronovost, P. A. Lipsett, D. Hobson, K. Earsing, J. E. Farley, S. Milanovich, E. Garrett-Mayer, B. D. Winters, and H. R. Rubin. 2004. "Eliminating

Catheter-Related Bloodstream Infections in the Intensive Care Unit." *Critical Care Medicine* 32 (10): 2014–20.

Berens, Michael J., and Bruce Japsen. 2002. "Patients Suffer as Agency Shields Troubled Hospitals." *Chicago Tribune*, November 10, 2002. http://articles.chicagotribune.com /2002-11-10/news/0211100494_1_joint-commission-accreditation-patient-deaths.

Berenson, A. 2008. "Weak Patchwork of Oversight Lets Bad Hospitals Stay Open." *New York Times,* December 8, 2008. http://www.nytimes.com/learning/students/pop /articles/08hospital.html.

Berridge, Virginia. 1999. *Health and Society in Britain since 1939.* Cambridge: Cambridge University Press.

Berry, Leonard, and Kent D. Seltman. 2008. *Management Lessons from Mayo Clinic: Inside One of the World's Most Admired Service Organizations.* New York: McGraw-Hill.

Berwick, Donald M. 1996. "A Primer on Leading the Improvement of Systems." *BMJ* 312 (7031): 619–22.

———. 2003. "Disseminating Innovations in Health Care." *Journal of the American Medical Association* 289 (15): 1969–75.

———. 2008. "A Transatlantic Review of the NHS at 60." *BMJ* 337: a838.

———. 2013. *Berwick Review into Patient Safety.* London: Department of Health.

Berwick, D. M., N. A. DeParle, D. M. Eddy, P. M. Ellwood, A. C. Enthoven, G. C. Halvorson, K. W. Kizer, E. A. McGlynn, U. E. Reinhardt, and R. D. Reischauer. 2003. "Paying for Performance: Medicare Should Lead." *Health Affairs* 22 (6): 8–10.

Bevan, Gwyn, and Christopher Hood. 2006. "What's Measured Is What Matters: Targets and Gaming in the English Public Health Care System." *Public Administration* 84 (3): 517–38.

Beveridge, William. 1942. *Social Insurance and Allied Services: Report.* London: HMSO.

Bewley, Helen. 2006. "Raising the Standard? The Regulation of Employment and Public Sector Employment Policy." *British Journal of Industrial Relations* 44 (2): 351–72.

Blair, Tony. 2002. *The Courage of Our Convictions: Why Reform of the Public Services Is the Route to Social Justice.* London: Fabian Society.

Blake, Mariah. 2010. "Dirty Medicine: How Medical Supply Behemoths Stick It to the Little Guy, Making America's Health Care System More Dangerous and Expensive." *Washington Monthly,* July–August 2010. http://www.washingtonmonthly.com /features/2010/1007.blake.html.

Blavin, Fredric, Adele Shartzer, Sharon K. Long, and John Holahan. 2015. "An Early Look at Changes in Employer-Sponsored Insurance under the Affordable Care Act." *Health Affairs* 34 (1): 170–77.

Blumenthal, David. 1999. "Health Care Reform at the Close of the 20th Century." *New England Journal of Medicine* 340 (24): 1916–20.

BMJ Editors. 2011. "Reaction: What They Say about the Health Bill." *BMJ* 342: d413.

Bosk, C. L., M. Dixon-Woods, C. A. Goeschel, and P. J. Pronovost. 2009. "Reality Check for Checklists." *Lancet* 374 (9688): 444–45.

Boukus, Ellyn, Alwyn Cassil, and Ann S. O'Malley. 2009. "A Snapshot of U.S. Physicians: Key Findings from the 2008 Health Tracking Study Physician Survey." *Data*

Bulletin, no. 35. Washington, DC: Center for Studying Health System Change. http://www.hschange.com/CONTENT/1078/.

Boyne, George A. 1999. *Managing Local Services: From CCT to Best Value*. London: Frank Cass.

British Medical Association. 1997. "An Outline History of the British Medical Association." British Medical Association. https://web.archive.org/web/20081122004118/http://www.bma.org.uk/ap.nsf/Content/BMAOutlineHistory.

Broadbent, Jane, and Richard Laughlin. 2005. "The Role of PFI in the UK Government's Modernisation Agenda." *Financial Accountability and Management* 21 (1): 75–97.

Brody, Jane E. 2008. "A Basic Hospital To-Do List Saves Lives." *New York Times*, January 22, 2008. http://www.nytimes.com/2008/01/22/health/22brod.html.

Brown, Gordon. 2003. "A Modern Agenda for Prosperity and Social Reform: Speech Made by the Chancellor of the Exchequer, Gordon Brown, to the Social Market Foundation at the Cass Business School, London." HM Treasury. http://www.hm-treasury.gov.uk/newsroom_and_speeches/press/2003/press_12_03.cfm.

Brownlee, Shannon. 2008. *Overtreated: Why Too Much Medicine Is Making Us Sicker and Poorer*. New York: Bloomsbury.

Buchan, J., and D. Evans. 2007. *Realising the Benefits? Implementing Agenda for Change*. London: King's Fund.

Buresh, Bernice, and Suzanne Gordon. 2006. *From Silence to Voice: What Nurses Know and Must Communicate to the Public*. 2nd ed. Ithaca, NY: Cornell University Press.

Cameron, David. 2008. "There Is Such a Thing as Society . . . and We Must Start to Value It." *Yorkshire Post*, 13 May 2008. http://www.yorkshirepost.co.uk/news/debate/columnists/david_cameron_there_is_such_a_thing_as_society_and_we_must_start_to_value_it_1_2500825.

Cameron, Sue. 2014. "David Nicholson—The Man Who Believed in Being Ruthless with the NHS." *The Telegraph*, 26 March 2014. http://www.telegraph.co.uk/news/nhs/10724504/David-Nicholson-the-man-who-believed-in-being-ruthless-with-the-NHS.html.

Care Quality Commission. 2014a. "Intelligent Monitoring: NHS Acute Hospitals," December 3, 2014. http://www.cqc.org.uk/content/intelligent-monitoring-nhs-acute-hospitals.

——. 2014b. "Intelligent Monitoring: NHS Acute Hospitals: Indicators and Methodology. Guidance to Support the December 2014 Intelligent Monitoring Update." London: Care Quality Commission.

Carpenter, Mick. 2000. "Between Elation and Despair: UNISON and the New Social Policy Agenda." In *Redefining Public Sector Unionism: UNISON and the Future of Trade Unions*, edited by Mike Terry, 193–213. London: Routledge.

Carvel, John. 2001. "Milburn Names the Worst Hospitals." *The Guardian*, September 26, 2001. http://www.theguardian.com/uk/2001/sep/26/johncarvel.

——. 2003. "Four of the 'Top' Hospitals Fall out of Running." *The Guardian*, July 16, 2003. http://society.guardian.co.uk/print/0,3858,4713083-106632,00.html.

Centers for Medicare and Medicaid Services. 2008. "Medicaid Managed Care Penetration Rates and Expansion Enrollment by State." Department of Health and Human Services, March 18, 2010. http://www.cms.gov/MedicaidDataSourcesGenInfo/05 _MdManCrPenRateandExpEnrll.asp.

Central Office of Information for the Ministry of Health. 1948. *The New National Health Service.* Pamphlet. London.

Chassin, Mark R., Jerod M. Loeb, Stephen P. Schmaltz, and Robert M. Wachter. 2010. "Accountability Measures—Using Measurement to Promote Quality Improvement." *New England Journal of Medicine* 363 (7): 683–88.

Clark, Paul F. 2013. "Health Care: Collective Bargaining's Growing Role in a Time of Transition." In *Collective Bargaining under Duress: Case Studies of Major U.S. Industries,* edited by Howard Stanger, Ann C. Frost, and Paul F. Clark, 119–64. Champaign, IL: Labor and Employment Relations Association.

Clarke, John, Sharon Gewirtz, and Eugene McLaughlin. 2000. "Reinventing the Welfare State." In *New Mangerialism, New Welfare?,* edited by John Clarke, Sharon Gewirtz, and Eugene McLaughlin, 1–26. London: Open University and Sage.

CMS Office of Public Affairs. 2012. "CMS Announces Data and Information Initiative." June 5, 2012. https://www.cms.gov/Research-Statistics-Data-and-Systems/Research /ResearchGenInfo/Downloads/OIPDA_Fact_Sheet.pdf.

Coalition of Kaiser Permanente Unions, and Kaiser Permanente. 2011. "UBT Basics." http://www.lmpartnership.org/ubt.

Collins, James W. 2010. "Statement by Capt. James W. Collins, Ph.D., M.S.M.E." May 11, 2010. http://www.hhs.gov/asl/testify/2010/05/t20100511a.html.

Commission for Health Improvement. 2003a. Clinical Governance Review: North Cumbria Acute Hospitals NHS Trust. London: Commission for Health Improvement.

Confederation of British Industry. 2006. *Working Together: Embedding Good Employment in Public Services.* London: Confederation of British Industry.

Connolly, Sheelah, Gwyn Bevan, and Nicholas Mays. 2010. *Funding and Performance of Healthcare Systems in the Four Countries of the UK before and after Devolution.* London: Nuffield Trust.

Conservative Party. 2009. "Stop Brown's NHS Cuts." http://www.conservatives.com /Campaigns/Stop_Browns_NHS_Cuts.aspx.

——. 2010. "Where We Stand: Health." http://www.conservatives.com/Policy/Where _we_stand/Health.aspx.

Cully, Mark, Stephen Woodland, Andrew O'Reilly, and Gill Dix. 1999. *Britain at Work: As Depicted by the 1998 Workplace Employee Relations Survey.* London: Routledge.

Cunningham, Robert, III, and Robert M. Cunningham Jr. 1997. *The Blues: A History of the Blue Cross and Blue Shield System.* DeKalb: Northern Illinois University Press.

Daley, Anthony, and Chris Howell. 1992–93. "The Transformation of Political Exchange." *International Journal of Political Economy* 22 (4): 3–16.

Dartmouth Institute for Health Policy and Clinical Practice. 2010. "Dartmouth Atlas of Health Care." Trustees of Dartmouth College. http://www.dartmouthatlas.org/.

Davies, Annette, and Ian Kirkpatrick. 1995. "Performance Indicators, Bureaucratic Control and the Decline of Professional Autonomy: The Case of Academic Librarians." In *The Politics of Quality in the Public Sector: The Management of Change*, edited by Ian Kirkpatrick and Miguel Martinez Lucio, 84–107. London: Routledge.

Davis, Karen, Karen Scott Collins, and Cynthia Morris. 1994. "Managed Care: Promise and Concerns." *Health Affairs* 13 (4): 178–85.

Davis, Karen, Kristof Stremikis, David Squires, and Cathy Schoen. 2014. *Mirror, Mirror on the Wall, 2014 Update: How the U.S. Health Care System Compares Internationally*. New York: Commonwealth Fund.

Dawson, Sandra, and Charlotte Dargie. 2002. "New Public Management: A Discussion with Special Reference to UK Health." In *New Public Management: Current Trends and Future Prospects*, edited by Kate McLaughlin, Stephen P. Osborne, and Ewan Ferlie, 34–56. London: Routledge.

Debley, Tom. 2009. *The Story of Dr. Sidney R. Garfield: The Visionary Who Turned Sick Care into Health Care*. Portland, OR: Permanente Press.

Democratic Policy Committee. 2010. "Archived Materials: The Patient Protection and Affordable Care Act as Passed." https://web.archive.org/web/20130313043147 /http://dpc.senate.gov/dpcdoc-sen_health_care_bill_archive_as_passed.cfm.

Department of Health. 2000a. *Improving Working Lives Standard*. London: Department of Health.

———. 2000b. *An Organisation with a Memory: Report of an Expert Group on Learning from Adverse Events in the NHS Chaired by the Chief Medical Officer*. London: The Stationery Office.

———. 2001a. *Building a Safer NHS for Patients: Implementing an Organisation with a Memory*. London: Department of Health.

———. 2001b. *NHS Performance Ratings: Acute Trusts*. London: Department of Health.

———. 2002a. *Delivering the NHS Plan: Next Steps on Investment, Next Steps on Reform*. London: The Stationery Office.

———. 2002b. *A Guide to NHS Foundation Trusts*. London: Department of Health.

———. 2002c. *NHS Performance Ratings: Acute Trusts, Specialist Trusts, Mental Health Trusts, 2001/02*. London: Department of Health.

———. 2003a. *Agenda for Change: Proposed Agreement*. Leeds: Department of Health.

———. 2003b. "Improving Working Lives." Department of Health, August 26, 2003. https://web.archive.org/web/20031229071348/http://www.doh.gov.uk/iwl/back ground.htm.

———. 2004a. *Agenda for Change: Final Agreement*. Leeds: Department of Health.

———. 2004b. *Standards for Better Health*. London: Department of Health.

Department of Health and Social Security. 1983. *Performance Indicators: National Summary for 1981*. London: Department of Health and Social Security.

DeWalt, D. A., J. Oberlander, T. S. Carey, and W. L. Roper. 2005–6. "Significance of Medicare and Medicaid Programs for the Practice of Medicine." *Health Care Financing Review* 27 (2): 79–90.

Dixon, Jennifer, Julian Le Grand, and Peter Smith. 2003. *Can Market Forces Be Used for Good?* London: King's Fund.

Donnelly, John. 2010. "Comparative Effectiveness Research (Updated)." *Health Affairs: Health Policy Briefs*, October 8, 2010. http://www.healthaffairs.org/healthpolicybriefs /brief.php?brief_id=28.

Dunn, Lindsey. 2014. "Toyota Is Not Lean," *Becker's Hospital Review: Daily Beat Blog*, September 24, 2014. http://www.beckershospitalreview.com/healthcare-blog/toyota-is -not-lean.html.

Eappen, Sunil, Bennett H. Lane, Barry Rosenberg, Stuart A. Lipstiz, David Sadoff, Dave Matheson, William R. Berry, Mark Lester, and Atul A. Gawande. 2013. "Relationship between Occurrence of Surgical Complications and Hospital Finances." *Journal of the American Medical Association* 309 (15): 1599–606.

Eaton, George. 2013. "The Pre-Election Pledges That the Tories Are Trying to Wipe from the Internet." *New Statesman*, November 13, 2013. http://www.newstatesman .com/politics/2013/11/pre-election-pledges-tories-are-trying-wipe-internet.

Edemariam, Aida, Jon Henley, and Homa Khaleeli. 2007. "A Picture of Health?" *The Guardian*, September 24, 2007. http://www.guardian.co.uk/film/2007/sep/24/health .politics.

Eisenberg, John M., Candice C. Bowman, and Nancy E. Foster. 2001. "Does a Healthy Health Care Workplace Produce Higher-Quality Care?" *Joint Commission Journal on Quality and Patient Safety* 27 (9): 444–57.

Emanuel, Ezekiel J. 2014. *Reinventing American Health Care: How the Affordable Care Act Will Improve Our Terribly Complex, Blatantly Unjust, Outrageously Expensive, Grossly Inefficient, Error Prone System*. New York: PublicAffairs.

Emanuel, Ezekiel J., and Linda L. Emanuel. 1996. "What Is Accountability in Health Care?" *Annals of Internal Medicine* 124 (2): 229–39.

Enthoven, Alain C. 1993. "The History and Principles of Managed Competition." *Health Affairs* 12 (Supplement 1): 24–48.

Esping-Andersen, Gøsta. *The Three Worlds of Welfare Capitalism*. Cambridge: Polity, 1990.

Fairbrother, Peter. 1996. "Workplace Trade Unionism in the State Sector." In *The New Workplace Trade Unionism*, edited by Peter Ackers, Chris Smith, and Paul Smith, 111–48. London: Routledge.

Foster, Andrew. 2002. *Inter-Professional Learning in the NHS*. Southampton: ASME and University of Southampton.

Gaffney, Adam. 2014. "The Twilight of the British Public Health System?" *Dissent* (Spring): 5–10.

Gaffney, Declan, Allyson M. Pollock, David Price, and Jean Shaoul. 1999. "The Private Finance Initiative: PFI in the NHS—Is There an Economic Case?" *BMJ* 319 (7202): 116–19.

Gaffney, F Andrew, Stephen W Harden, and Rhea Seddon. 2005. *Crew Resource Management: The Flight Plan for Lasting Change in Patient Safety*. Marblehead, MA: HC Pro.

Gates, Alexandra, Robin Rudowitz, and Jocelyn Guyer. 2014. *An Overview of Delivery System Reform Incentive Payment (DSRIP) Waivers*. Menlo Park, CA: Henry J. Kaiser Family Foundation.

Gawande, Atul. 2007. "The Checklist." *New Yorker,* December 10, 2007. http://www
.newyorker.com/magazine/2007/12/10/the-checklist.

Gawande, Atul. 2009a. *The Checklist Manifesto: How to Get Things Right.* New York:
Metropolitan Books.

———. 2009b. "The Cost Conundrum: What a Texas Town Can Teach Us about Health
Care." *New Yorker,* June 1, 2009. http://www.newyorker.com/magazine/2009/06/01
/the-cost-conundrum.

Giaimo, Susan. 2001. "Who Pays for Health Care Reform?" In *The New Politics of the
Welfare State*, edited by Paul Pierson, 334–67. Oxford: Oxford University Press.

Giaimo, Susan, and Philip Manow. 1999. "Adapting the Welfare State: The Case of
Health Care Reform in Britain, Germany and the United States." *Comparative Political Studies* 32 (8): 967–1000.

Gilmer, Todd, and Richard Kronick. 2001. "Calm before the Storm: Expected Increase
in the Number of Uninsured Americans." *Health Affairs* 20 (6): 207–10.

Gittell, Jody Hoffer. 2009. *High Performance Healthcare: Using the Power of Relationships
to Achieve Quality, Efficiency and Resilience.* New York: McGraw-Hill.

Gittell, Jody Hoffer, Kathleen M Fairfield, Benjamin Bierbaum, William Head, Robert
Jackson, Michael Kelly, Richard Laskin, Stephen Lipson, John Siliski, and Thomas
Thornhill. 2000. "Impact of Relational Coordination on Quality of Care, Postopera-
tive Pain and Functioning, and Length of Stay: A Nine-Hospital Study of Surgical
Patients." *Medical Care* 38 (8): 807–19.

Givan, Rebecca. 2010–11. "The Maimonides Medical Center Model: Reducing Conflict
through Mutual Respect and Resolving It through Mediation." *Dispute Resolution
Journal* 65 (4): 11, 54–6.

Givan, Rebecca Kolins. 2005. "Seeing Stars? Performance Management and Human
Resources in the National Health Service." *Personnel Review* 34 (6): 634–47.

Givan, Rebecca Kolins, Ariel Avgar, and Mingwei Liu. 2010. "Having Your Cake and
Eating It Too? The Relationship between HR Management and Organizational Performance in Healthcare." *Advances in Industrial and Labor Relations* 17 (1): 31–67.

Givan, Rebecca Kolins, and Stephen Bach. 2007. "Workforce Responses to the Creeping
Privatization of the UK National Health Service." *International Labor and Working
Class History* 71 (1): 133–53.

Glennerster, Howard. 2000. *British Social Policy since 1945.* 2nd ed. Oxford: Black-
well.

GMB. 2002a. "PFI: The 'Retention of Employment' Policy for PFI in NHS. Briefing
Note for GMB by Public Service Insight." https://web.archive.org/web/20021226193648
/http://www.gmb.org.uk/docs/ViewADocument.asp?ID=483&CatID=62.

———. 2002b. "Who Are the Real Wreckers?" GMB [Web site]. http://www.gmb.org.uk
/docs/ViewADocument.asp?ID=626&CatID=62.

Gold, Jenny. 2014. "FAQ on ACOs: Accountable Care Organizations, Explained,"
April 16, 2014. http://kaiserhealthnews.org/news/aco-accountable-care-organization
-faq/.

Goldacre, M., and K Griffin. 1983. *Performance Indicators: A Commentary on the Literature.* Oxford: University of Oxford Unit of Clinical Epidemiology.

Gordon, Suzanne. 2005. *Nursing against the Odds.* Ithaca, NY: Cornell University Press.

———. 2009. "Institutional Obstacles to RN Unionization: How 'Vote No' Thinking Is Deeply Embedded in the Nursing Profession." *WorkingUSA* 12 (2): 279–97.

Gordon, Suzanne, John Buchanan, and Tanya Bretherton. 2008. *Safety in Numbers: Nurse-to-Patient Ratios and the Future of Health Care.* Ithaca, NY: Cornell University Press.

Gordon, Suzanne, Patrick Mendenhall, and Bonnie Blair O'Connor. 2012. *Beyond the Checklist: What Else Health Care Can Learn from Aviation Teamwork and Safety:* Ithaca, NY: Cornell University Press.

Gottschalk, Marie. 2000. *The Shadow Welfare State: Labor, Business, and the Politics of Health-Care in the United States.* Ithaca, NY: Cornell University Press.

Green, T. P. 2007. "Management Skills of Intensivists Influence Outcomes in Pediatric Intensive Care Units." *Pediatric Critical Care Medicine* 8 (6): 587.

Green-Pedersen, Christoffer, and Markus Haverland. 2002. "The New Politics and Scholarship of the Welfare State." *Journal of European Social Policy* 12 (1): 43–51.

Grimshaw, Damian, Steve Vincent, and Hugh Willmott. 2002. "Going Privately: Partnership and Outsourcing in UK Public Services." *Public Administration* 80 (3): 475–502.

Gubb, James. 2009. "Have Targets Done More Harm Than Good in the English NHS? Yes." *BMJ* 338: a3130.

Gunningham, Neil, and Joseph Rees. 1997. "Industry Self-Regulation: An Institutional Perspective." *Law & Policy* 19 (4): 363–414.

Hacker, Jacob S. 1997. *The Road to Nowhere: The Genesis of President Clinton's Plan for Health Security.* Princeton, NJ: Princeton University Press.

Hales, B. M., and P. J. Pronovost. 2006. "The Checklist—a Tool for Error Management and Performance Improvement." *Journal of Critical Care* 21 (3): 231–35.

Hall, Peter A., and David W. Soskice, eds. 2001. *Varieties of Capitalism: The Institutional Foundations of Comparative Advantage.* Oxford: Oxford University Press.

Ham, Chris, and Paul Zollinger-Read. 2012. "What Are the Lessons from the USA for Clinical Commissioning Groups in the English National Health Service?" *Lancet* 379 (9811): 189–91.

Hansard (Commons). 2002a. "House of Commons Hansard Debates for 14 Nov 2002." London: UK Parliament.

———. 2002b. "House of Commons Hansard Debates for 30 Jan 2002." London: UK Parliament.

Hariri, S., K. J. Bozic, C. Lavernia, A. Prestipino, and H. E. Rubash. 2007. "Medicare Physician Reimbursement: Past, Present, and Future." *Journal of Bone and Joint Surgery* 89 (11): 2536–46.

Haynes, Alex B., Thomas G. Weiser, William R. Berry, Stuart R. Lipsitz, Abdel-Hadi S. Breizat, E. Patchen Dellinger, Teodoro Herbosa, Sudhir Joseph, Pascience L. Kibatala, Marie Carmela M. Lapitan, Alan F. Merry, Krishna Moorthy, Richard K. Reznick, Bryce Taylor, and Atul A. Gawande. 2009. "A Surgical Safety Checklist to Reduce Morbidity and Mortality in a Global Population." *New England Journal of Medicine* 360 (5): 491–99.

Healthcare Commission. 2004. "Performance Indicators for the Star Ratings 2003/04: Key Targets and Performance Indicators for Acute & Specialist Trusts." London: Healthcare Commission.

Heaton, Norma, Bob Mason, and Joe Morgan. 2002. "Partnership and Multi-Unionism in the Health Service." *Industrial Relations Journal* 33 (2): 112–26.

Heinrich, Janet. 2000. *Occupational Safety: Selected Cost and Benefit Implications of Needlestick Prevention Devices for Hospitals.* Washington, DC: US General Accounting Office.

Henry J. Kaiser Family Foundation. 2005. "Employer Health Benefits 2005 Annual Survey." The Henry J. Kaiser Family Foundation. http://www.kff.org/insurance/7315/sections/ehbs05-5-1.cfm.

———. 2009. "Total HMO Enrollment." Henry J. Kaiser Family Foundation. http://www.statehealthfacts.org/comparetable.jsp?ind=348&cat=7&sub=85&yr=71&typ=1&sort=a.

———. 2010. Survey of People Who Purchase Their Own Insurance. Menlo Park, CA: Henry J. Kaiser Family Foundation.

———. 2015a. "State Health Facts: Health Insurance Coverage of the Total Population." Henry J. Kaiser Family Foundation. http://kff.org/other/state-indicator/total-population/.

———. 2015b. "State Health Facts: Providers and Service Use." Henry J. Kaiser Family Foundation. http://kff.org/state-category/providers-service-use/.

———. 2015c. Total HMO Enrollment July 2013.

Herszenhorn, David M., and Sheryl Gay Stolberg. 2009. "Health Plan Opponents Make Voices Heard." *New York Times*, August 3, 2009. http://www.nytimes.com/2009/08/04/health/policy/04townhalls.html.

HM Treasury. 2014. *Private Finance Initiative Projects: 2014 Summary Data.* London: HM Treasury.

Hunter, David J. 2002. "A Tale of Two Tribes: The Tension between Managerial and Professional Values." In *Hidden Assets: Values and Decision-Making in the NHS,* edited by Bill New and Julia Neuberger, 61–78. London: King's Fund.

Hurley, Robert E., Bradley C. Strunk, and Justin S. White. 2004. "The Puzzling Popularity of the PPO." *Health Affairs* 23 (2): 56–68.

Huselid, Mark A. 1995. "The Impact of Human Resource Management Practices on Turnover, Productivity, and Corporate Financial Performance." *Academy of Management Journal* 38 (3): 635–72.

Ichniowski, Casey, Kathryn Shaw, and Giovanna Prennushi. 1997. "The Effects of Human Resource Management Practices on Productivity: A Study of Steel Finishing Lines." *American Economic Review* 87 (3): 291–313.

Iglehart, John K. 2001. "The Centers for Medicare and Medicaid Services." *New England Journal of Medicine* 345 (26): 1920–24.

Immergut, Ellen. 1992. *Health Politics: Interests and Institutions in Western Europe.* Cambridge: Cambridge University Press.

Irvine, Donald. 2001. "The Changing Relationship Between the Public and the Medical Profession: The Lloyd Roberts Lecture." Royal Society of Medicine. http://www.gmc-uk.org/news/lloyd_roberts_lecture.htm.

Jacoby, Sanford M. 1997. *Modern Manors: Welfare Capitalism since the New Deal.* Princeton, NJ: Princeton University Press.

James, John T. 2013. "A New, Evidence-based Estimate of Patient Harms Associated with Hospital Care." *Journal of Patient Safety* 9 (3): 122–28.

Joint Commission. 2008. "New Hospital Deeming Law and the Joint Commission." *The Joint Commission: Perspectives* 28 (9): 1, 10.

———. 2011. "Facts about the Unannounced Survey Process." The Joint Commission. http://www.jointcommission.org/assets/1/18/Unannounced_Survey_Process_9_12.pdf.

———. 2012a. *Improving Patient and Worker Safety: Opportunities for Synergy, Collaboration and Innovation.* Oakbrook Terrace, IL: Joint Commission.

———. 2012b. "Joint Commission History," Joint Commission. https://web.archive.org/web/20140611231602/http://www.jointcommission.org/assets/1/6/Joint_Commission_History.pdf.

Jones, Kathleen. 1994. *The Making of Social Policy in Britain 1830–1990.* 2nd ed. London: Athlone Press.

Josie King Foundation. 2007. [2012] Josie King Foundation [Web site]. http://www.josieking.org/.

Jost, Timothy Stoltzfus. 1983. "The Joint Commission on Accreditation of Hospitals: Private Regulation of Health Care and the Public Interest." *Boston College Law Review* 24 (4): 835–923.

———. 1994. "Medicare and the Joint Commission on Accreditation of Healthcare Organizations: A Healthy Relationship?" *Law and Contemporary Problems* 57 (4): 15–45.

Jowett, Paul, and Margaret Rothwell. 1988. *Performance Indicators in the Public Sector.* London: Macmillan.

Julius, DeAnne. 2008. *Public Services Industry Review: Understanding the Public Services Industry: How Big, How Good, Where Next?* Department for Business, Enterprise and Regulatory Reform. http://webarchive.nationalarchives.gov.uk/20121212135622/http://www.bis.gov.uk/files/file46965.pdf.

Kaiser Permanente, and the Coalition of Kaiser Permanente Unions. 2010. "2010 National Agreement." Labor Management Partnership. http://www.lmpartnership.org/what-is-partnership/national-agreements/2010-national-agreement.

———. 2012. "2012 National Agreement." Labor Management Partnership. http://www.lmpartnership.org/2012-national-agreement.

Katz, Harry Charles, and Owen Darbishire. 2000. *Converging Divergences: Worldwide Changes in Employment Systems.* Ithaca, NY: Cornell University Press.

Kerr, Clark, John T. Dunlop, Frederick Harbison, and Charles. A. Myers. 1964. *Industrialism and Industrial Man: The Problems of Labor and Management in Economic Growth.* 2nd ed. New York: Oxford University Press.

Kleiner, Morris M. 2006. *Licensing Occupations: Ensuring Quality or Restricting Competition?* Kalamazoo, MI: W. E. Upjohn Institute for Employment Research.

Kochan, Thomas A., Adrienne E. Eaton, Robert B. McKersie, and Paul S. Adler. 2009. *Healing Together: The Labor-Management Partnership at Kaiser Permanente.* Ithaca, NY: Cornell University Press.

Kochan, Thomas A., Harry Charles Katz, and Robert B. McKersie. 1986. *The Transformation of American Industrial Relations.* New York: Basic Books.

Kohn, Linda T., Janet Corrigan, and Molla S. Donaldson. 2000. *To Err Is Human: Building a Safer Health System*. Washington, DC: National Academy Press.

Koppel, R., J. P. Metlay, A. Cohen, B. Abaluck, A. R. Localio, S. E. Kimmel, and B. L. Strom. 2005. "Role of Computerized Physician Order Entry Systems in Facilitating Medication Errors." *Journal of the American Medical Association* 293 (10): 1197–203.

Koppel, Ross, and Suzanne Gordon, eds. 2012. *First, Do Less Harm: Confronting the Inconvenient Problems of Patient Safety*. Ithaca, NY: Cornell University Press.

Kovner, Christine. 2001. "The Impact of Staffing and the Organization of Work on Patient Outcomes and Health Care Workers in Health Care Organizations." *Joint Commission Journal on Quality and Patient Safety* 27 (9): 458–68.

Kronick, Richard, and Todd Gilmer. 1999. "Explaining the Decline in Health Insurance Coverage, 1979–1995." *Health Affairs* 18 (2): 30–47.

Kuttner, Robert. 1998. "Must Good HMOs Go Bad? First of Two Parts: The Commercialization of Prepaid Group Health Care." *New England Journal of Medicine* 338 (21): 1558–63.

Labour Party. 2001. *Ambitions for Britain: Labour's Manifesto 2001*. London: Labour Party.

Lazes, Peter, Maria Figueroa, and Liana Katz. 2012. "How Labor-Management Partnerships Improve Patient Care, Cost Control, and Labor Relations: Case Studies of Fletcher Allen Health Care, Kaiser Permanente, and Montefiore Medical Center," Cornell University. https://www.ilr.cornell.edu/sites/ilr.cornell.edu/files/Case-Studies-Final-3-7-2012.pdf.

Lee, Fred. 2004. *If Disney Ran Your Hospital: 9 1/2 Things You Would Do Differently*. Bozeman, MT: Second River Healthcare Press.

Le Grand, Julian. 2003. *Motivation, Agency and Public Policy*. Oxford: Oxford University Press.

Light, Donald W. 2003. "Universal Health Care: Lessons from the British Experience." *American Journal of Public Health* 93 (1): 25–30.

Lindrooth, R. C., G. J. Bazzoli, J. Needleman, and R. Hasnain-Wynia. 2006. "The Effect of Changes in Hospital Reimbursement on Nurse Staffing Decisions at Safety Net and Nonsafety Net Hospitals." *Health Services Research* 41 (3): 701–20.

Lister, John. 2003. *The PFI Experience: Voices from the Frontline*. London: UNISON.

Mares, Isabella. 2000. "Strategic Alliances and Social Policy Reform: Unemployment Insurance in Comparative Perspective." *Politics and Society* 28 (2): 223–44.

Markus, Anne Rossier, Ellie Andres, Kristina D West, Nicole Garro, and Cynthia Pellegrini. 2013. "Medicaid Covered Births, 2008 through 2010, in the Context of the Implementation of Health Reform." *Women's Health Issues* 23 (5): e273–80.

Martinez Lucio, Miguel, and Robert MacKenzie. 1999. "Quality Management: A New Form of Control?" In *Employee Relations in the Public Services: Themes and Issues*, edited by Susan Corby and Geoff White, 156–74. London: Routledge.

Maynard, Alan. 1991. "Developing the Health Care Market." *Economic Journal*: 1277–86.

Maynard, Alan, and Karen Bloor. 2003. "Do Those Who Pay the Piper Call the Tune?" *Health Policy Matters* 8: 1–8.

McLaughlin, Kate, Stephen P. Osborne, and Ewan Ferlie, eds. 2002. *New Public Management: Current Trends and Future Prospects*. London: Routledge.

McNeil Jr, R., and R. E. Schlenker. 1975. "HMOs, Competition, and Government." *Milbank Memorial Fund Quarterly. Health and Society* 53 (2): 195–224.

Meckstroth, T. W. 1975. " 'Most Different Systems' and 'Most Similar Systems': A Study in the Logic of Comparative Inquiry." *Comparative Political Studies* 8 (2): 132–57.

Menendez, J. B. 2010. "The Impetus for Legislation Revoking the Joint Commission's Deemed Status as a Medicare Accrediting Agency." *JONA's Healthcare Law, Ethics and Regulation* 12 (3): 69–76.

Merrifield, Nicola. 2015. "Unions Make Link between Guidance Suspension and Staffing Costs." *Nursing Times*, June 4, 2015.

Michael, Douglas C. 1995. "Federal Agency Use of Audited Self-Regulation as a Regulatory Technique." *Administrative Law Review* 47 (2): 171–253.

Michaels, R. K., M. A. Makary, Y. Dahab, F. J. Frassica, E. Heitmiller, L. C. Rowen, R. Crotreau, H. Brem, and P. J. Pronovost. 2007. "Achieving the National Quality Forum's "Never Events": Prevention of Wrong Site, Wrong Procedure, and Wrong Patient Operations." *Annals of Surgery* 245 (4): 526–32.

Milkman, Ruth, and Stephanie Luce. 2014. *The State of the Unions 2014: A Profile of Organized Labor in New York City, New York State, and the United States.* New York: Murphy Institute, City University of New York.

Miller, M. R., P. Pronovost, M. Donithan, S. Zeger, C. Zhan, L. Morlock, and G. S. Meyer. 2005. "Relationship between Performance Measurement and Accreditation: Implications for Quality of Care and Patient Safety." *American Journal of Medical Quality* 20 (5): 239–52.

Moffett, Maurice L., Robert O. Morgan, and Carol M. Ashton. 2005. "Strategic Opportunities in the Oversight of the U.S. Hospital Accreditation System." *Health Policy* 75 (1): 109–15.

Monbiot, George. 2000. *Captive State: The Corporate Takeover of Britain.* London: Macmillan.

Moncrieff, A., and E. Lee. 2012. "The Positive Case for Centralization in Healthcare Regulation: The Federalism Failures of the ACA." *Kansas Journal of Law and Public Policy* 20: 266–92.

Moran, Michael. 2000. "Understanding the Welfare State: The Case of Health Care." *British Journal of Politics and International Relations* 2 (2): 135–60.

Morgan, Philip, and Christopher Potter. 1995. "Professional Cultures and Paradigms of Quality in Health Care." In *The Politics of Quality in the Public Sector: The Management of Change*, edited by Ian Kirkpatrick and Miguel Martinez Lucio, 166–89. London: Routledge.

National Nurses United. 2015. "National Campaign for Safe RN-to-Patient Staffing Ratios." National Nurses United [Web site]. http://www.nationalnursesunited.org/issues/entry/ratios.

National Workforce Taskforce, and HR Directorate. 2002. *HR in the NHS Plan.* London: Department of Health.

Nelson, Sioban. 2001. *Say Little, Do Much: Nurses, Nuns, and Hospitals in the Nineteenth Century.* Philadelphia: University of Pennsylvania Press.

NHS. 2015. "NHS Choices." http://www.nhs.uk/pages/home.aspx.

NHS Employers. 2014. "Agenda for Change Pay." NHS Employers, June 10, 2014. http://www.nhsemployers.org/agendaforchange.

NHS Executive. 2000. *Quality and Performance in the NHS: NHS Performance Indicators.* London: NHS Executive.

Nuffield Trust. 2013. *Rating Providers for Quality: A Policy Worth Pursuing?* London: Nuffield Trust.

Panitch, Leo, and Colin Leys. 1997. *The End of Parliamentary Socialism.* New York: Verso.

Parks, James. 2011. "California Nurses Win Improvements in Tentative Kaiser Deal." *AFL-CIO Now Blog,* January 11, 2011. https://web.archive.org/web/20110119143255/http://blog.aflcio.org/2011/01/11/california-nurses-win-improvements-in-tentative-kaiser-deal/.

Patient-Centered Outcomes Research Institute. 2014. "About US," PCORI, October 6, 2014. http://www.pcori.org/about-us.

Pawlson, L. Gregory, and Margaret E. O'Kane. 2002. "Professionalism, Regulation, and the Market: Impact on Accountability for Quality of Care." *Health Affairs* 21 (3): 200–7.

Pear, Robert. 2009. "Health Care Spending Disparities Stir a Fight." *New York Times,* June 8, 2009. http://www.nytimes.com/2009/06/09/us/politics/09health.html.

Peedell, Clive. 2011. "Further Privatisation Is Inevitable under the Proposed NHS Reforms." *BMJ* 342: d2996.

Performance Indicator Group. 1987. *Acute Hospital Services.* London: Department of Health and Social Security.

Pew Charitable Trusts, and MacArthur Foundation. 2014. "State Employee Health Plan Spending: An Examination of Premiums, Cost Drivers, and Policy Approaches." http://www.pewtrusts.org/en/research-and-analysis/reports/2014/08/state-employee-health-plan-spending.

Pierson, Paul. 1994. *Dismantling the Welfare State? Reagan, Thatcher and the Politics of Retrenchment.* Cambridge: Cambridge University Press.

———. 1996. "The New Politics of the Welfare State." *World Politics* 48 (2): 143–79.

Piore, Michael J., and Charles. F. Sabel. 1984. *The Second Industrial Divide: Possibilities for Prosperity.* New York: Basic Books.

Pizzorno, Alessandro. 1978. "Political Exchange and Collective Identity in Industrial Conflict." In *The Resurgence of Class Conflict in Western Europe since 1968,* vol. 2, edited by Colin Crouch and Alessandro Pizzorno, 277–98. London: MacMillan.

Pollitt, Christopher, Stephen Harrison, George Dowswell, Sonja Jerak-Zuiderent, and Roland Bal. 2010. "Performance Regimes in Health Care: Institutions, Critical Junctures and the Logic of Escalation in England and the Netherlands." *Evaluation* 16 (1): 13–29.

Pollock, Allyson M. 2004. *NHS plc: The Privatisation of Our Health Care.* London Verso.

———. 2015. "Will Politicians Be Architects or Destroyers of the NHS?" *Lancet* 385 (9974): 1171–72.

Pollock, Allyson M., Matthew Dunnigan, Declan Gaffney, Alison Macfarlane, and F. Azeem Majeed. 1997. "What Happens When the Private Sector Plans Hospital Services for the NHS: Three Case Studies under the Private Finance Initiative." *BMJ* 314 (7089): 1266–71.

Pollock, Allyson M, and Peter Roderick. 2015. "Why the Queen's Speech on 19 May Should Include a Bill to Reinstate the NHS in England." *BMJ* 350: h2257.

Power, Michael. 1997. *The Audit Society: Rituals of Verification*. Oxford: Oxford University Press.

Pronovost, P., D. Needham, S. Berenholtz, D. Sinopoli, H. Chu, S. Cosgrove, B. Sexton, R. Hyzy, R. Welsh, and G. Roth. 2006. "An Intervention to Decrease Catheter-Related Bloodstream Infections in the ICU." *New England Journal of Medicine* 355 (26): 2725–32.

Pronovost, Peter, and Eric Vohr. 2010. *Safe Patients, Smart Hospitals: How One Doctor's Checklist Can Help Us Change Health Care from the Inside Out*. New York: Hudson Street Press.

Propper, Carol, and Deborah Wilson. 2003. "The Use and Usefulness of Performance Measures in the Public Sector." *Oxford Review of Economic Policy* 19 (2): 250–67.

Public Administration Select Committee. 2002. *The Public Service Ethos: Seventh Report of Session 2001–02*. vol. 1. London: Stationery Office.

———. 2003. *Select Committee on Public Administration Fifth Report*. London: United Kingdom Parliament.

Purcell, John. 2004. *The HRM-Performance Link: Why, How and When Does People Management Impact on Organisational Performance?* John Lovett Memorial Lecture 2004. Limerick: University of Limerick.

Ratcliffe, R. L. 2009. "Re-engineering Hospital Accreditation." *Clinical Governance* 14 (4): 315–35.

Riley-Smith, Ben. 2014. "NHS Chief Executive Calls on Next Government Not to Implement Top-Down Reorganisation of Service." *The Telegraph,* October 23, 2014. http://www.telegraph.co.uk/news/health/news/11181731/NHS-chief-executive-Simon -Stevens-calls-on-next-government-not-to-implement-top-down-reorganisation-of -service.html.

Robinson, James C. 2003. "The Curious Conversion of Empire Blue Cross." *Health Affairs* 22 (4): 100–18.

Rogers, A. E., W. T. Hwang, L. D. Scott, L. H. Aiken, and D. F. Dinges. 2004. "The Working Hours of Hospital Staff Nurses and Patient Safety." *Health Affairs* 23 (4): 202–12.

Rosenthal, Elisabeth. 2013. "American Way of Birth, Costliest in the World." *New York Times* June 30, 2013. http://www.nytimes.com/2013/07/01/health/american-way-of -birth-costliest-in-the-world.html.

Rosenthal, Meredith B. 2007. "Nonpayment for Performance? Medicare's New Reimbursement Rule." *New England Journal of Medicine* 357 (16): 1573–75.

Royal College of Nursing. 2000. *An RCN Guide to the Private Finance Initiative*. London: Royal College of Nursing.

———. 2003. "Agenda for Change." Royal College of Nursing. https://www.rcn.org.uk /support/pay_and_conditions/agendaforchange.

Sager, Ira. 2013. "Where the Growth Is in Management Consulting." *Bloomberg Business: The Management Blog,* June 13, 2013. http://www.bloomberg.com/bw/articles/2013-06-13/where-the-growth-is-in-management-consulting.

Sanger-Katz, Margot. 2014. "Is the Affordable Care Act Working? Has the Percentage of Uninsured People Been Reduced?" *New York Times,* October 27, 2014. http://www.nytimes.com/interactive/2014/10/27/us/is-the-affordable-care-act-working.html.

Schilling, Lisa, James W. Dearing, Paul Staley, Patti Harvey, Linda Fahey, and Francesca Kuruppu. 2011. "Kaiser Permanente's Performance Improvement System, Part 4: Creating a Learning Organization." *Joint Commission Journal on Quality and Patient Safety* 37 (12): 532–43.

Schrage, Michael. 1995. "Accreditation Becomes Battleground for Defining Quality Health Care." *Washington Post,* April 21, 1995. http://www.washingtonpost.com/archive/business/1995/04/21/accreditation-becomes-battleground-for-defining-quality-health-care/af3b99e1-1ceb-4b0c-9ff4-74fe868e85cc/.

Schyve, P. M. 2000. "The Evolution of External Quality Evaluation: Observations from the Joint Commission on Accreditation of Healthcare Organizations." *International Journal for Quality in Health Care* 12 (3): 255–58.

Scott, R. Douglas, II, and Division of Healthcare Quality Promotion. 2009. *The Direct Medical Costs of Healthcare-Associated Infections in US Hospitals and the Benefits of Prevention.* CS200891-A. Atlanta: Division of Healthcare Quality Promotion National Center for Preparedness, Detection, and Control of Infectious Diseases, Centers for Disease Control and Prevention.

Shannon, R. P., D. Frndak, N. Grunden, J. C. Lloyd, C. Herbert, B. Patel, D. Cummins, A. H. Shannon, P. H. O'Neill, and S. J. Spear. 2006. "Using Real-Time Problem Solving to Eliminate Central Line Infections." *Joint Commission Journal on Quality and Patient Safety* 32 (9): 479–87.

Shifrin, Tash. 2003. "Private Firm Takes over NHS Hospital." *The Guardian,* September 1, 2003. http://www.theguardian.com/society/2003/sep/01/hospitals.nhs.

Shortell, Stephen M., Waters, Teresa. M., Clarke Kenneth W. B., Budetti, Peter B. 1998. "Physicians as Double Agents: Maintaining Trust in an Era of Multiple Accountabilities." *Journal of the American Medical Association* 280 (12): 1102–8.

Silberner, Joanne. 2011. "Head of Major HMO Sees Openings for Accountable Care Organizations—The KHN Interview." Kaiser Health News, July 25, 2011. http://khn.org/news/halvorson-q-and-a-kaiser-permanente-accountable-care-organizations/.

Skocpol, Theda. 1995. "The Rise and Resounding Demise of the Clinton Plan." *Health Affairs* 14 (1): 66–85.

Smee, Clive. 2002. "Improving Value for Money in the United Kingdom National Health Service: Performance Measurement and Improvement in a Centralised System." In *Measuring Up: Improving Health System Performance in OECD Countries,* edited by Peter Smith, 57–85. Paris: OECD.

Smith, Richard. 2002. "Take Back Your Mink, Take Back Your Pearls." *BMJ* 325 (7372): 1047–48.

Southwick, Frederick S. 2013. "Losing My Leg to a Medical Error." *New York Times,* February 19, 2013. http://www.nytimes.com/2013/02/20/opinion/losing-my-leg-to-a-medical-error.html.

Stark, Hon. Fortney Pete. 1998. "Why the Joint Commission on Accrediting Health-care Organizations (JCAHO) Must Do Better." *Congressional Record* 144 (145): E2139–140.

Starr, Paul. 1982. *The Social Transformation of American Medicine*. New York: Basic Books.

——. 1994. *The Logic of Health-Care Reform: Why and How the President's Plan Will Work*. Rev. ed. New York: Whittle/Penguin.

Steinbrook, Robert. 2009. "Easing the Shortage in Adult Primary Care—Is It All about Money?" *New England Journal of Medicine* 360 (26): 2696–99.

Stevens, Simon. 2004. "Reform Strategies for the English NHS." *Health Affairs* 23 (3): 37–44.

Swenson, Peter. 2002. *Capitalists against Markets: The Making of Labor Markets and Welfare States in the United States and Sweden*. Oxford: Oxford University Press.

Swenson, Peter, and Scott Greer. 2002. "Foul Weather Friends: Big Business and Health Care Reform in the 1990s in Historical Perspective." *Journal of Health Politics Policy and Law* 27 (4): 605–38.

Tailby, Stephanie. 2005. "Agency and Bank Nursing in the UK National Health Service." *Work, Employment and Society* 19 (2): 369–89.

Thiebaud, Lorriane. 2000. "Testimony of Lorraine Thiebaud, RN on Behalf of the Service Employees International Union (SEIU), AFL-CIO." *Federal News Service,* June 22, 2000, http://lobby.la.psu.edu/047_Needlestick_Injuries/Congressional_Hearings/Testimony/H_Edu_Workforce_Prot_062200_5.htm.

Thorlby, Ruth. 2009. "A Healthy Debate? The US and English Health Systems." King's Fund, June 2, 2009. http://www.kingsfund.org.uk/blog/2009/08/healthy-debate-usa-english-health-system-difference.

Timmins, Nicholas. 2012. *Never Again?, Or, The Story of the Health and Social Care Act 2012: A Moderne [sic] Drama in Five Incompleted Acts*. London: King's Fund.

Toynbee, Polly. 2013. "Simon Stevens, New Head of NHS England, Is in for a Rude Awakening." *The Guardian,* October 25, 2013. http://www.theguardian.com/commentisfree/2013/oct/25/simon-stevens-nhs-england-rude-awakening.

UNISON. 2002a. "Composite 2: Public Services." London: Motion at Labour Party Conference.

——. 2002b. "PFI: Failing Our Future. A UNISON Audit of the Private Finance Initiative." London: UNISON. https://www.yumpu.com/en/document/view/8817765/pfi-failing-our-future-unison.

——. 2013. "UNISON Responds to Appointment of Simon Stevens as NHS Chief Executive." *UNISON News,* October 24, 2013. https://www.unison.org.uk/news/article/2013/10/unison-responds-to-appointment-of-simon-stevens-as-nhs-chief-executive/.

University of Michigan Center of Excellence in Public Health Workforce Studies. 2013. *Public Health Workforce Enumeration, 2012*. Ann Arbor: University of Michigan.

Urbina, Ian. 2009. "Beyond Beltway, Health Debate Turns Hostile," *New York Times,* August 7, 2009. http://www.nytimes.com/2009/08/08/us/politics/08townhall.html.

US Bureau of Labor Statistics. 2009. "Occupational Outlook Handbook, 2010–11 Edition, Physicians and Surgeons," Office of Occupational Statistics and Employment Projections. https://web.archive.org/web/20110728091313/http://www.bls.gov/oco/ocos074.htm.

———. 2010. "Career Guide to Industries, 2010–11 Edition: Healthcare," Office of Occupational Statistics and Employment Projections. https://web.archive.org/web/20120113164022/http://www.bls.gov/oco/cg/cgs035.htm.

———. 2014. "Occupational Outlook Handbook, 2014–15 Edition, Physicians and Surgeons." US Department of Labor. http://www.bls.gov/ooh/healthcare/physicians-and-surgeons.htm.

———. 2015. "Industries at a Glance: Health Care and Social Assistance: NAICS 62." US Department of Labor. http://www.bls.gov/iag/tgs/iag62.htm.

US Department of Health and Human Services, Health Resources and Services Administration, and National Center for Health Workforce Analysis. 2014. *The Future of the Nursing Workforce: National- and State-Level Projections, 2012–2025.* Rockville, MD.

US Health Resources and Services Administration. 2010. "HRSA Study Finds Nursing Workforce is Growing and More Diverse." US Department of Health and Human Services, March 17, 2010. http://www.hrsa.gov/about/news/pressreleases/100317_hrsa_study_100317_finds_nursing_workforce_is_growing_and_more_diverse.html.

US Government Accountability Office. 2004. *Medicare: CMS Needs Additional Authority to Adequately Oversee Patient Safety in Hospitals: Report to Congressional Requesters.* GAO-04-850. Washington, DC: US Government Accountability Office.

US House of Representatives. 2000. *OSHA's Compliance Directive on Bloodborne Pathogens and the Prevention of Needlestick Injuries: Hearing before the Subcommittee on Workforce Protections of the Committee on Education and the Workforce, House of Representatives, 106th Cong., Second Session, Hearing Held in Washington, DC, June 22, 2000.* Washington, DC: US Government Printing Office.

US Occupational Safety and Health Administration (OSHA), US Department of Labor. 2008. "Healthcare Facilities." Safety and Health Topics. http://www.osha.gov/SLTC/healthcarefacilities/index.html.

———. 2013. "Safe Patient Handling." Safety and Health Topics. http://www.osha.gov/SLTC/healthcarefacilities/safepatienthandling.html.

US Office of Personnel Management. 2014. "OPM Announces 2015 Federal Employees Health Benefits Program Premium Rates." News release, October 7, 2014. https://www.opm.gov/news/releases/2014/10/opm-announces-2015-federal-employees-health-benefits-program-premium-rates/.

US Senate, Committee on Health, Education, Labor and Pensions, Subcommittee on Employment and Workplace Safety. 2010. "Subcommittee Hearing: Safe Patient Handling and Lifting Standards for a Safer American Workforce." 111th cong., 2nd sess., May 11, 2010, US Senate. http://www.help.senate.gov/hearings/hearing/?id=6a53554d-5056-9502-5da3-4d68bc6b9f48.

Vest, Joshua R., and Larry D. Gamm. 2009. "A Critical Review of the Research Literature on Six Sigma, Lean and StuderGroup's Hardwiring Excellence in the United

States: The Need to Demonstrate and Communicate the Effectiveness of Transformation Strategies in Healthcare." *Implementation Science* 4: 35–35.

VitalSmarts. 2008. "Crucial Conversations Improves Patient Safety at Brooklyn Hospital by Building a Culture of Respect." VitalSmarts. http://www.vitalsmarts.com/case studies/maimonides/.

Vize, Richard. 2014. "What Impact Do Regulators Have on the NHS?" *The Guardian*, December 11, 2014. http://www.theguardian.com/healthcare-network/2014/dec/11 /impact-regulators-nhs-care-quality-commission.

Wachter, Bob. 2011. "Top-Down vs. Bottom-Up." *The Health Care Blog,* September 28, 2011. http://thehealthcareblog.com/blog/2011/09/28/top-down-vs-bottom-up/.

Waddington, Jeremy, and Allan Kerr. 1999. "Membership Retention in the Public Sector." *Industrial Relations Journal* 30 (2): 151–65.

Walker, Stuart R., and Rachel M. Rosser. 1993. *Quality of Life Assessment: Key Issues in the 1990s: Key Issues in the 1990s.* Dordrecht, Netherlands: Springer Science + Business Media.

Wang, Dora, et al. 2015. "US and British Health Specialists Support the NHS." *The Guardian,* May 3, 2015. http://www.theguardian.com/politics/2015/may/03/us-and -british-health-specialists-support-the-nhs.

Webster, Charles. 2002. *The National Health Service: A Political History.* 2nd ed. Oxford: Oxford University Press.

Weiner, B. J., J. A. Alexander, S. M. Shortell, L. C. Baker, M. Becker, and J. J. Geppert. 2006. "Quality Improvement Implementation and Hospital Performance on Quality Indicators." *Health Services Research* 41 (2): 307–34.

Weiner, S. M. 1977. " 'Reasonable Cost' Reimbursement for Inpatient Hospital Services under Medicare and Medicaid: The Emergence of Public Control." *American Journal of Law and Medicine* 3 (1): 1–47.

West, Michael A., Carol Borrill, Jeremy Dawson, Judy Scully, Matthew Carter, Stephen Anelay, Malcolm Patterson, and Justin Waring. 2002. "The Link between the Management of Employees and Patient Mortality in Acute Hospitals." *Internal Journal of Human Resource Management* 13 (8): 1299–310.

Willett, Vita. 2013. "Getting Personal about Workplace Safety: How One Leader Engages Her Team and Others to Get Results." Labor Management Partnership, June 13, 2013. http://www.lmpartnership.org/stories-videos/getting-personal-about-workplace -safety.

Wintour, Patrick. 2002. "Political Route Map That Led to Dead End." *The Guardian,* April 27, 2002. http://politics.guardian.co.uk/fiveyears/story/0,11899,706100,00.html.

Womack, James P., Daniel T. Jones, and Daniel Roos. 1991. *The Machine That Changed the World: How Japan's Secret Weapon in the Global Auto Wars Will Revolutionize Western Industry.* New York: HarperPerennial.

Woolf, S. H. 2004. "Patient Safety Is Not Enough: Targeting Quality Improvements to Optimize the Health of the Population." *Annals of Internal Medicine* 140 (1): 33–36.

Workforce and Facilities Team. 2015. "NHS Workforce Statistics—February 2015, Provisional Statistics." Health and Social Care Information Centre, May 21, 2015. http:// www.hscic.gov.uk/catalogue/PUB17529.

Working Group on Indicators for the Community Health Services. 1988. *Report of the Working Group on Indicators for the Community Health Services.* London: Department of Health and Social Services.

Zwerdling, Daniel. 2015. "Despite High Rates of Nursing Injuries, Government Regulators Take Little Action." *National Public Radio*, March 24, 2015. http://www.npr.org /2015/03/24/394823592/despite-high-rates-of-nursing-injuries-government-regulators -take-little-action.

INDEX

CPSIA information can be obtained at www.ICGtesting.com
Printed in the USA
BVOW03*2050190816

459592BV00002B/9/P